What Others Are Saying about *Th*
also by Phil and A...

"*The 90-Day Fitness Challenge* is a wonderful compilation of the principles, anecdotes, and information that not only helped to change the lives of my friends, Phil and Amy Parham, but can serve to change the lives of its readers as well. From their DREAM principle to the daily mini-challenges and tips, along with the combination of faith principles, inspirational quotes, and noteworthy statistics, Phil and Amy provide guidance for anyone looking to get on the path to a healthy lifestyle."

—**BILL GERMANAKOS**, winner, Season 4 of *NBC's The Biggest Loser*

"*The 90-Day Fitness Challenge* is a great read for those desiring to lose weight and keep God at the center. Having watched Phil and Amy work out at D1, I believe their testimony will motivate and inspire people to desire to better themselves. I have been around the fitness industry a long time and have a strong passion for overall wellness. It is awesome to experience Phil and Amy sharing a similar passion!"

—**WILL BARTHOLOMEW**, president and CEO,
D1 Sports Training and Therapy

"Phil and Amy Parham prove there are no quick fixes, but in *The 90-Day Fitness Challenge*, they show how in a brief period of time you can lay the foundation for a lifetime of healthy habits."

—**BRANDI KOSKIE**, DietsInReview.com

"Phil and Amy Parham inspired me on *The Biggest Loser*, and they will inspire you to reach your goals. This book covers aspects of health that so many others leave out. I was excited to get to the next chapter!"

—**DANNY CAHILL**, winner, Season 8 of *NBC's The Biggest Loser*

"The first book that I've ever read that clearly spells out the right steps to take to gain a healthy lifestyle. Phil and Amy Parham have taken the guesswork out of the equation. Apply these principles and in 90 days your DREAM will be a reality."

—**ROB DEMPSEY**, morning radio DJ and multisport athlete

"It takes a special kind of courage to face your personal demons, and an even greater courage to accept that many of them exist as a result of your bad choices. The ultimate courage is to right those wrongs. Phil and Amy Parham have done just that, and their book will inspire many of us to do the same."

—**BILL ELLIS**, morning radio host, "Ellis and Bradley Morning Show"

"Being on *The Biggest Loser* was one of the most significant times in my Christian life. God designed and desires us to be spiritually and physically healthy, and the impact on our lives is huge. Phil and Amy Parham are the only ones to have put into writing what so many former contestants now know—that weight loss, pursuing health, and becoming the person God intended us to be is not just an exercise program, but a faith journey as well. As a pastor and weight-loss group leader, I love that *The 90-Day Fitness Challenge* is a complete program, tying together amazing teaching and resources on changing to a healthy lifestyle while honoring and involving our Creator. This is THE book to get for individuals or groups looking to change their lives for the long term!"

—REV. MATTHEW MCNUTT, contestant,
Season 3 of *NBC's The Biggest Loser*

"Phil and Amy Parham's *The 90-Day Fitness Challenge* is more than your typical diet book. They don't just *tell* you how to achieve long-lasting change in your life; they *show* you how to do it. Their story is inspiring, and their enthusiasm for good health and fitness is contagious. If you're looking for a practical program that can help you transform your life through realizing the critical connection between the physical and the spiritual, then *The 90-Day Fitness Challenge* may be exactly what you're looking for."

—JULIE HADDEN, first runner-up and biggest female loser,
Season 4 of *NBC's The Biggest Loser*;
author, *Fat Chance: Losing the Weight, Gaining My Worth*

"If you've tried every diet out there and are finally open to adopting a new way of life that gives you a real chance for success, look no further than Phil and Amy Parham's *The 90-Day Fitness Challenge*. Chock-full of motivation, sound advice, and doable actions that will set you up for a lifetime of success, it's a must-have guide for health and happiness!"

—DEVIN ALEXANDER, host of *Healthy Decadence* (FitTV) and
author of the *New York Times* bestselling *Biggest Loser* cookbooks

"Amy and Phil Parham will help you understand that nutrition and fitness is a lifetime journey...not a sprint."

—DR. RICK KATTOUF II, host of *Rx Nutrition*
DVDs and author of *Forever Fit*

The
Amazing
Fitness
Adventure
for Your Kids

AMY PARHAM
PHIL PARHAM

HARVEST HOUSE PUBLISHERS

EUGENE, OREGON

Cover design by Dugan Design Group, Bloomington, Minnesota

Cover photo © Martin Barraud / OJO Images / Getty Images

Published in association with Fedd & Company, Inc. Literary Agency

Readers are advised to consult with their physician or other medical practitioner before implementing the suggestions that follow. This book is not intended to take the place of sound professional medical advice or to treat specific maladies. Neither the author nor the publisher assumes any liability for possible adverse consequences as a result of the information contained herein.

The Biggest Loser **is not associated with this book or any of the views or information contained in this book.**

THE AMAZING FITNESS ADVENTURE FOR YOUR KIDS
Copyright © 2011 by Phil and Amy Parham
Published by Harvest House Publishers
Eugene, Oregon 97402
www.harvesthousepublishers.com

Library of Congress Cataloging-in-Publication Data
   Parham, Phil, 1966-
   The Amazing Fitness Adventure for your Kids / Phil and Amy Parham.
      p. cm.
   ISBN 978-0-7369-3921-8 (pbk.)
   ISBN 978-0-7369-4189-1 (eBook)
   1. Physical fitness for children.   2. Children—Health and hygiene.   I. Parham, Amy, 1967-
II. Title.   III. Title: Ninety-day fitness challenge for your kids.
   RJ133.P37 2011
   613.7'042—dc22
                                                              2010046524

Contents

Acknowledgments

From Amy

Above all, we thank our Lord and Savior Jesus Christ. Without Him we wouldn't be able to live this beautiful dream called life.

This book is dedicated to our three boys, Austin, Pearson, and Rhett. They are each so unique and special in their own ways, and we are honored and blessed to have been chosen to be their parents. No matter what mountains I climb or what goals I reach, my greatest accomplishment will be if I raised them to be the men that God created them to be.

From Phil

This is our third book! I almost cannot believe we have accomplished so much in such a short time. I need to tell my beautiful wife, Amy, once again how much I love and appreciate her. She is a gift from God to me. She took this project on her back and ran with it. I also want my kids to know I love them and pray they live the future of their dreams. This book is also dedicated to the children all over our great nation. We wish them a limitless, meaningful, and healthy life.

Amy and I both want to acknowledge AJ, Esther, Jim, Dina, Monique, and all the wonderful people in our Harvest House family. Without you we couldn't be who we are. We love and appreciate you all.

Introduction

Amy's Story

Six years ago, I was lying on my couch, gazing through an opening in the ceiling that led to the attic. My eyes slowly became fixated on a wooden beam. I began to wonder: What would it feel like if I hung myself? Could the beam support my weight? How would I do it? My downward spiral into a deep depression had reached the bottom. I felt completely hopeless and began to contemplate a permanent way out. How in the world did I allow myself to get to this point?

In four years, I had given birth to three sons (Austin was born on March 24, 1995; Pearson on April 30, 1997; and our baby Rhett on October 22, 1999) and had gained 70 pounds. My body and spirit sagged under the pressure of the extra weight. In 2003, Rhett was diagnosed with autism. As any mother who has high hopes and dreams for her children, I struggled with the diagnosis and dedicated much of my time and energy into finding ways to "fix" Rhett. I was physically exhausted and emotionally drained. I coped by binge eating every night, which made me put on more and more weight. At the same time, my husband's business had collapsed, and we found ourselves under incredible financial pressure.

Every day felt like hell on earth. I would make myself get out of bed each morning, even though I didn't feel like it. One day I was driving down the road and I was praying, as I always did, for some guidance on how to find a miracle cure for Rhett because I couldn't accept that he wasn't going to be "normal." In the depths of my spirit, I heard God say, "Amy, you are not perfect and I love you. Why does Rhett have to be perfect for you to love him?" Instantly I felt a burden lift off my shoulders as I realized that if I would just love my little boy and trust God, He would take care of my son. This was the first step of my journey to get my life back on track.

Though the road was unbelievably long and hard at times, eventually the financial part of our lives and the challenges of having a child with autism began to straighten out. I knew that our weight was the last frontier to conquer. One night in 2008, having reached clinical obesity at 229 pounds, I was sitting on the sofa eating ice cream, crying, and watching *The Biggest Loser*. I suddenly decided to look on NBC.com to see what the process was for getting on the show.

A few months later, on Valentine's Day weekend, Phillip and I were in Atlanta for the auditions. Though we were hopeful, we didn't hear anything from the network until two and a half months later. From the moment we were contacted until we were actually on the show was a whirlwind. Before we knew it, Phillip and I were on a plane to Los Angeles as finalists, though we were not yet promised a slot on the show. The next week, Bob Harper, one of the show's fitness trainers, surprised us at our home to announce that out of 300,000 applicants, we were chosen for Season 6 of *The Biggest Loser*. Tears flowed down my face, and I remember thinking that this was the last piece of the puzzle to getting our lives back. There was no turning back.

Phil's Story

Even though I was an overweight child, I never let it stop me from becoming a success in business and being able to support my family. In 2004, however, my mortgage broker business went to pieces after my business partner left. It was a shock to my ego and a crushing blow to our bank accounts. My family lost not only our luxurious lifestyle, but also our security. For the first time in my life, I was at a loss about what to do. My weight slowly began to creep up the scales, but I wasn't paying attention to it that much. I was too busy trying to formulate a plan on how to get my family out of debt. My health was the last thing on my mind.

I had no choice but to turn this devastating situation over to God about the same time my wife also surrendered. We knew that with Him, there had to be a way out of the pressure. Slowly but surely our lives started to turn around. My wife and I found new careers in real estate. We became the top sales agents, selling over 60 homes in our first year. We also found a new therapy for Rhett that helped him improve his language and behavior. While we were both feeling more inspired and motivated,

Amy and I were still too busy with our family and new careers to give much thought to our personal health. Pushing 40, constantly feeling out of breath and struggling to maintain my energy level, I knew it was only a matter of time before I had to do something about my weight. The one area I had casually ignored my whole life would now become my battleground.

I was at my heaviest, a staggering 340 pounds, when my wife took a step toward change and applied for both of us to be contestants on *The Biggest Loser*. There we began a new chapter of transforming our physical bodies—the only part of our lives that was holding us back from fulfilling all of our dreams. In only seven months, we together lost over 250 pounds, putting me at a trim 180 pounds and my wife Amy at a svelte 124 pounds. We still have one of the highest percentages of weight loss of any couple in *The Biggest Loser*'s history. Though we were on the show for only two and a half months, the entire process actually lasted seven months—two and a half months was spent on "the ranch," the place we went to for the program's highly intense exercise and nutrition regimen, and the rest of the time was spent at home getting ready for the live finale seven months later.

Today

We've maintained our healthy weight as we've incorporated permanent lifestyle changes we learned on *The Biggest Loser* into our family's lifestyle. We've seen dramatic changes with our kids. Pearson, who was slightly overweight, lost pounds just by us eliminating sodas, snacks, and sweets from our home. All our kids became more active by participating in family hikes and 3K races. Austin joined the cross-country team. Pearson decided to start training to play football. And Rhett learned how to ride his bike for the first time.

We have spent time away from the show as a chance to share with others the power of transforming health. The most life-changing lesson we've learned on our journey is that our success is only a small part of the big picture to inspire others. By living out our dreams, we are dedicated to helping others also live out their dreams.

When we got home from the ranch, we not only witnessed an outpouring of love and support, but we also got asked a lot of questions about how we changed our health so dramatically. Our good friend William Hayes suggested we get local sponsorship and plan an event to instruct and encourage others to take the same journey and to provide answers to the questions of weight loss. So we took another step of faith and created the "90-Day Fitness Challenge," a program designed to help others lose weight and gain health in 90 days based on how we did it ourselves.

With much running around, making countless phone calls, and tending to last-minute details, we put together our first event in less than two weeks at LivN Nsidout Wellness Complex in Simpsonville, South Carolina, on January 7, 2009. Almost a thousand people showed up from five states. We were blown away at how magical the event turned out, especially since it was organized at the last minute. When we saw how many people wanted to learn more about healthy living and losing weight, we put a mailing list together and sent out daily emails to these folks. We offered tips, encouragement, and pointed them in the right direction to better living. As weeks and months went by, the reports we got back were astounding. We received email after email from people who lost weight guided by what they learned in the "90-Day Fitness Challenge." Not only did the pounds drop, but many of these wonderful people experienced other life changes—some quit smoking, some mended their marriages, and others gained the courage to pursue lifelong dreams.

At the end of 90 days, we had a finale party sponsored by several local businesses. It was amazing to see the transformation of the people who had attended the initial event three months earlier. Those who had come to that first meeting depressed were now excited. Those who were unhealthy were now healthy. Those who felt tired, sluggish, and unmotivated were now energized, inspired, and motivated. It was an emotional and powerful experience for us, far beyond what words can say. These beautiful people reminded us of our own transformation.

We knew that God wanted to get this message out to more than just those folks, so we got involved with online communities, churches, corporations, and other organizations all across the United States.

Not only that, but in the last year, we especially were encouraged to motivate families. We have seen the dangers of childhood obesity and the damage excess weight can cause kids and their families. We witnessed the effects of poor nutrition in our own family before our transformation.

We believe in the power of families to create a home that is healthy, happy, and fit. We have a heartfelt empathy for families who want to transform their unhealthy, sedentary lifestyles into positive, healthy ones, and we want to walk with them on their journey.

We have been blessed to be a part of giving people a chance to reclaim their life by bettering their health. And we have been blessed by seeing many wonderful changes in our own family as we have taken the path to better health. We hope to do the same for you with this book, which we have based on our first book, *The 90-Day Fitness Challenge*.

The Amazing Fitness Adventure for Your Kids will show you how to transform your life and live your dreams of being a healthy, happy, and more fit family. This book is divided into two parts.

Part 1 includes seven chapters that teach fundamentals of being healthy, such as

- how important it is to dream of having a healthy family
- why it's necessary to monitor our children's health and weight
- how we must lead the journey as parents
- how to eat better and exercise more
- how to maintain good health in the middle of life's busyness
- how to use basic life-changing principles to jump-start your way into the "90-Day Challenge."

In Part 2 of the book, we will walk together with you through 90 days of your family's journey to better health by offering inspiration, motivation, and practical life skills through our daily challenge. These challenges should be read together as a family.

We will include stories from our own lives, weight-management skills and tips learned from our experience on the show, and motivational weight-loss stories of those who have been inspired by our success.

This book is not a diet plan. It is about making a lifestyle change. This book is relevant to families wherever they fall on the health barometer. If you or your children are not overweight and you are fairly healthy, this book is still a great tool to maintain those good habits in your home (and you'll be surprised what more you can learn!). If you or your children need some help making better health choices, this book will teach you how you can make those better choices. And if you want your children to enter adulthood equipped with solid nutrition and fitness habits, this book is for you.

The Amazing Fitness Adventure for Your Kids teaches parents not only how to raise healthy kids, it also provides a roadmap of the ultimate rewards and possibilities that come from sharing a healthy lifestyle together. This process will build stronger and healthier kids and closer-knit families. And isn't that what we all really want?

Do you want your family to have more energy? Do you want your family to be more active? Do you want your family to feel better? Do you want your family to be motivated? Challenged? Inspired?

We know you do, and now is the time!

Are you ready to get started?

Part 1

Back to the Basics

1

Dream Big!

W hen Phillip and I returned home from *The Biggest Loser* ranch, we experienced the beginning of an amazing physical transformation. All of our friends, families, and fans of the show had a slew of questions for us. "How did you do it?" "What was it like?" "Was it hard to do?" But two questions we were repeatedly asked stuck out in our mind—"Wasn't it hard to leave your kids while going on the show?" and "Where were your kids during that time?"

At the time we were chosen as contestants for *The Biggest Loser*, Austin was 12 years old, Pearson was 10, and Rhett was 8. Trust me, it wasn't easy to leave them for three months. Phillip and I gave a lot of thought to the impact our departure would have on them before we even considered trying out for the show. Although we competed to better our health, we knew that in doing so, we would better the physical, emotional, and even spiritual health of our family as a whole. Ultimately, in many ways, we did the show for our kids.

Phillip's sister, Joan, was a major influence in persuading us to try out for *The Biggest Loser*, and she even offered to watch our boys during the time we were away. If it weren't for her, we probably would have never even considered undertaking the opportunity. Joan had been concerned about our health for quite some time. She was also a big fan of the show and was the first person who encouraged me to watch it. I was resistant at first because I didn't know the premise behind it. I initially believed it was a show that made fun of fat people, but I quickly discovered I was wrong. *The Biggest Loser* isn't simply a reality TV show where contestants compete against each other to lose weight. I like to think of it as a powerful tool that helps forever change the lives of individuals and families.

During our absence, our boys were cared for by Joan and her husband, John, who have three boys similar in age to ours. My children and their family quickly formed a Brady Bunch of sorts. The cousins shared a tight-knit bond, and many wonderful memories were created that my boys still talk about today. We were so fortunate to have Joan and John—as well as my parents, sisters Allyson and Donna, and loving neighbors—who made tremendous personal sacrifices in order for Phillip and me to have the opportunity to transform our lives for the better.

Dreaming Big for Our Family

While we were gone, I felt incomplete because I missed our boys terribly. You can't imagine how difficult it was to know that my husband and I wouldn't be in contact with them for an undetermined amount of time. Our saving grace was knowing our family was taking good care of our children, and they were in the best hands we could have asked for. During the show, Phillip and I were also fortunate to win a particular contest where the prize was a phone call to our boys and a 24-hour visit home to see them.

However challenging it was for us to be away from our boys for so long, we knew the reward was greater than the price we were paying. This was a time we had to sacrifice for our family and take care of ourselves so we could become better role models for our kids. Not only that, but we also had to take care of our physical health so we could stick around for them.

Phillip and I were morbidly obese, and at the rate we were going, we had some serious health risks. I especially thought of Rhett and his autism and his need for special care. He needed us around for a long time. If Phillip or I had a heart attack or suffered from a life-threatening ailment because of our obesity, what would happen to our boys? Nobody wants to think about those kinds of things, but we had no choice. Phillip and I had to face some hard facts in order to reevaluate our priorities and make positive change.

Being on the show was a step in the direction of dreaming big for our family. We wanted the best for us and for them. Sometimes dreaming big as a parent means taking time for ourselves. That can be a hard thing for some folks. Many parents fear that when they focus on themselves, their children will deem them selfish and become resentful or spiteful. But this is not true when you commit to making changes that ultimately benefit your entire family. (I'm not talking about spending money reserved for paying bills on a fancy car you don't need or not helping your child with homework because you have to get your nails done. I'm talking about making good choices that will exact positive change.)

Phillip and I were not the best role models when it came to eating right and exercising regularly, but it was time to change all those bad habits into good ones. And it took time for us apart from our children to get the ball rolling. When we came back from *The Biggest Loser* ranch, we found that our family was reenergized by the changes we had made in our lives. When we changed, our children wanted to change too. They wanted to follow our example and dream big for their own lives. This meant making changes in their health.

Making Changes

There was no doubt that we had to do an about-face with many of the lifestyle habits in our home. The biggest area that needed a major overhaul was nutrition. Our boys got an introductory course in good health when family members took care of them. I believe this prepared them for our return and transformation. Joan and John are excellent parents and provide a great example of what a fit and healthy family should be. While our boys were under their care, Joan kept a close watch on what they ate and limited their snacks. They weren't used to this in the Parham household.

Before our weight-loss experience, we had poor eating habits as a family. We ate fast food almost every day, and our meals outside of the drive-thru were usually processed foods. Convenience always trumped nutritional content. We were (and still are) a busy family on a budget, so it made the most sense to eat fast and cheap. I thought I was doing my kids a favor. At least that's what the TV commercials led me to believe. I'm sure you've seen the advertisements for boxed meals that require only one or two "real" ingredients. They picture a doting mom, happy kids, and a warm meal that took no time to whip up. It was cheap, easy, and tasted great. This was something I could do, I thought. Look at me, I'm a good mom!

For most of my life, I bought into this lie hook, line, and sinker. I didn't realize that providing my children with meals and snacks low in nutrition was negatively affecting their energy levels, mental focus, and overall health. I didn't realize that not feeding them with foods designed to fuel their body meant they would not function at their best. I didn't realize that fatty, greasy, and salty foods would not just make them feel bad in the long run, but would increase their chances of getting sick later on. After being on the show, Phillip and I understood how critical it is to teach our kids good nutrition habits and provide a solid framework for good health that will ultimately help them be successful in life.

As a working mother, I also carried a lot of guilt for not spending enough time with my sons. One way I soothed my guilt was by giving them sugary or salty treats like cookies, candy, and chips. I worked a lot to help provide financially for my family, and I thought I had to "make it up" to my kids. I wanted to be one of the moms you see on TV who greets her children from school wearing fashionable clothes, sporting perfectly styled hair, and holding out a plate of freshly made chocolate chip cookies that melt in your mouth. I was no such mother. On the days I couldn't be home when they returned from school, I left them a bag of packaged cookies they could snack on in my absence.

You might relate. Do you feel that you're not giving enough time or energy to your children and ease your guilt by giving them forbidden snacks? If you miss a baseball practice or dance recital, do you make it up by letting your son or daughter eat something they really shouldn't? Are you so busy doing the million things most of us do that focusing on good nutrition is just not a priority?

Do you not even have the time to think about how poor eating habits will affect your children 5, 10, or 20 years from now? Maybe you think of illnesses such as heart disease and diabetes as "grown up" problems. I know I did. I thought my kids had plenty of time before they had to worry about those issues. I figured they needed to grow up first, and then they could pay attention to what they ate and what kind of exercise they got. This is poor thinking.

I believe this comes from the mind-set that going on a "diet" is reserved for adults. Now, dieting is not the answer for children or for adults. Dieting denotes something that you go on and come off of. It's about restricting food and eating in a way that is temporary and can't be continued for life. We should think about being healthy and fit. We need to permanently change our habits to healthy ones. This applies to adults and children. The truth is, kids who have healthy habits growing up have a better chance of sustaining a healthy lifestyle as they get older.

We need to make small changes every day that can add up to a new life. Whether it's saying yes to natural foods and no to processed foods or going for a walk instead of watching TV, the little things we do accumulate into a future worth having. A future that is healthy and makes you feel good inside and out. A future worth dreaming about.

We need to encourage our children that when they are healthy, they gain a better life. They can do more things and they can think more clearly. They will have more energy to be active. They will have better mental focus and get better grades. They will feel stronger and not get sick as much.

It's a win-win situation. Gaining health is a positive process that will help them succeed in whatever they do. It will give them the confidence to live as if the sky is the limit and to know that their dreams are within reach.

When Dreams Die

Our children don't need poor health to stand in the way of a great life. They need to give their dreams a chance to blossom. They need to be unencumbered from feeling tired, sluggish, or moody—things that come from making poor health choices—in order to dream big. Their ability to "go for it" should never be restricted by their size, physical-fitness level, or because of a negative self-image.

Childhood should be a time of dreaming, yet here's a sobering reality. Childhood obesity has become so prevalent that it has tempered our children's potential to dream big. This condition has locked them in a prison built with forks and spoons. Poor health prevents them from attempting new things.

As a parent, I know this may be a tough pill for you to swallow, especially if you have allowed bad lifestyle choices to rule your home. But don't be discouraged. This is not the time to question your parenting skills, feel sorry for yourself, or give up. This is a time for change!

Today you can commit to creating a healthy lifestyle for your family.

Today you can make sure your child's future is not limited by poor eating or exercising habits. Today you can lead your children in this "Challenge" to become healthier. And today, you can embark on a new adventure to witness your children gain confidence, feel better about themselves, and dream big.

When I was a girl, I struggled with weight. I gave up on many dreams because of that battle. Here's one I'll never forget. Like most teenage girls, I wanted to be a cheerleader. I remember feeling so out of place during the first tryout because I was the chubbiest girl there. My confidence level hit rock bottom, and I dropped out before I even had the chance to try out. I had many similar experiences.

I was always picked last when teams were selected for gym. I never raised my hand in class because I was afraid the other kids would laugh at me. I shied away from any physical activity at school because I was so big and doing the simplest things exhausted me. Because of my weight, my self-esteem suffered. I wasn't carefree and having fun. I was miserable.

I became comfortable with not taking risks and not taking a stab at doing new things; it was safer not to even try. Sadly, this mind-set stayed along for the ride as I grew up and entered adulthood. It was a tough mentality to break, but through losing weight and working on my emotional and mental health, I was able to break free from harmful thinking. And as I like to say, I am not a fat girl anymore; I'm a fit girl.

You too have the power to change. You can make better decisions that afford your children the chance to dream big, create a future full of possibilities, and shine.

Don't get wrapped up in the guilt of feeling you haven't done enough for your children or haven't helped them make the right choices. Guilt is a wasted emotion. Guilt will keep you emotionally paralyzed so that you won't do anything to change your circumstances. Guilt will not change a single thing, but here's the light at the end of the tunnel—taking a step in the right direction will.

Taking the First Step

Decisions pave the way to making dreams come true. Making the right decisions will change the course of your life and the life of your children. When Phillip and I decided to go on *The Biggest Loser*, we had to move heaven and earth to make it happen. We had to sell our cars and major household items so that my family would have enough money to operate while we were gone. I had to leave my children. I had to endure the physical, emotional, and mental process, which was grueling at times. None of these things were fun or convenient. None of these things were easy. But the payoff was amazing and totally worth it.

Former Boy Scout administrator Forest Witcraft once wrote, "A hundred years from now it will not matter what my bank account was, the sort of house I lived in, or the kind of car I drove. But the world may be different because I was important in the life of a boy." When I worked as an early childhood director at my church, I printed those words on bookmarks and gave them to all the volunteers who worked with me. The bookmarks were one way I reminded them that their sacrifice would last long after they were gone.

As a parent, you need to constantly remind yourself of that same truth. What you sacrifice today when it comes to your children will still be paying off long after you leave this earth. You have the power to affect their future for the better. You have the power to influence what their legacy will be. You have the power to commit to bettering the health of your household. I know you are ready to make this change because you are already reading this book. I am confident you want the best for your children and that you want to see their dreams come true.

Yes, sometimes dreaming big dreams requires overcoming big challenges. Don't worry. We will help you along the way. Believe me, we have had to work our way through many challenges that could have stopped us cold. Our book will equip you with knowledge, tools, and inspiration so you can move any mountains that may stand in your way of creating a healthy home.

Think about what dreaming big as a family looks like to you. Maybe it's as simple as eating better and exercising more. Maybe you want to lose a few pounds to have more energy to play with your daughter. Maybe you want to improve your health because you just got diagnosed with diabetes or another serious disease. Maybe you want to incorporate fitness into your family life and start running 5Ks together. Whatever it is, dreaming big means improving the quality of your family life. And that will guarantee a brighter future.

Today, take the first step and commit to making your children's health a priority so that you can see their dreams come true. It only takes a simple decision to change your life and your future.

Walk with us on this journey and let's dream big together!

2

Face the Facts

Dreaming is fun, isn't it? It is such a big first step in your new adventure of gaining better health. After we dust off our box of hidden dreams, the next critical step is to face some facts. And some of them might not be pretty.

You are reading this book because you believe you and your family will benefit from this fitness challenge. This means some poor habits are in place that you need to change. You might acknowledge that *you* need to be healthier, but for whatever reason you give your kids more slack. You might be thinking one or more of the following thoughts:

- *Why do I need to concern myself with what my kids eat and how much exercise they get?*

- *Is it really so bad that they eat fast food? They get to be kids only once, after all! Let them live a little, right? Since when did a little fast food hurt anybody?*

- *What's wrong with letting my kids play video games, play on the computer, and watch television after school? They work hard all day. Shouldn't they be able to veg out in front of the TV to unwind? Everyone needs a little break.*

- *What's the harm in having a little baby fat? They'll eventually grow out of it. I mean, really, what's the big deal?*

Prior to our health transformation, I used to be defensive when it came to our family's health habits. So if you're feeling the same way, I understand.

The Facts

Before we deal with some of these questions, let's get some facts straight.

Childhood obesity is an epidemic. It has almost tripled in the last 30 years. The 2008 "Facts for Families" report published by the American Academy of Child and Adolescent Psychiatry remarked that an estimated 17 percent of children and adolescents ages 2–19 years are obese. This unhealthy weight gain in our children stems from poor nutrition and inactivity.

A child is considered obese when her weight is at least 10 percent higher than what is recommended for her height and body type. Studies have shown that an obese child between the ages of 10 and 13 has an 80 percent chance of becoming an obese adult.

Though these facts are eye-opening and disturbing, the trend can be stopped. Childhood obesity is preventable if we work on changing to a healthy lifestyle. If an obese child has a greater chance of becoming an obese adult, you can see what a big deal it is for parents to model and implement healthy habits in the home as early as possible.

Contrary to what many people believe, obesity and weight gain do not come solely from genetics or biology. Most of our unhealthy habits come from behaviors we learn in our culture and in our home. And sadly, many of these behaviors are harmful to our health—from the plethora of fast-food restaurants, to the indulgence of processed foods, to the inactivity caused by spending too much time watching TV or playing video games.

Creating a healthy lifestyle in the home may be a challenge, especially if you have not maintained good nutrition or fitness goals for a long time, but it is doable and it is imperative if you want to raise a healthy family.

Priorities! Priorities! Priorities!

Give me a break, Phil and Amy. I'm a busy parent. I can't do everything perfectly. Nobody's perfect!

This might be your thought as you find yourself in the fast-food restaurant drive-thru for the fifth time this week. Sure, you'd rather be like Betty Crocker and put a hot meal on the table every night, but really, who does that anymore? Who has the time?

So many of us justify our actions when it comes to our kids' diet and exercise habits because we are simply overwhelmed with all of our other responsibilities. Most of us have more than enough to do during the day. We work full- or part-time, spend time with our kids doing homework, manage their after-school activities, clean our house, make time for our friends, meet our spouse's needs, volunteer in the schools or community, go to church. And that's just a few items in the long laundry list (oh, did I mention laundry?) most of us have.

It's much easier to go to the drive-thru after school for a quick meal or pick up a pizza after baseball practice than to sit home cooking. And I know how easy it is, when you do find an afternoon that's free, to stick your kids in front of the TV or put a video controller in their hand while you take a nap or watch a movie instead of going to the park as a family. The thought of adding more things, like exercise and making your own snacks and meals, to our ever-growing to-do list is exhausting.

Trust me, I know that feeling. I am no Harriet Nelson and my life definitely isn't a TV Land show. As a mother of three boys, I am well aware of how stressful raising children can be. There never seems to be enough time to do everything you need to do. I have gone to bed many nights knowing I had so many things left undone and feeling guilty that I let my kids down (again). I have juggled all the balls that you have to juggle as a working mom raising a family, and I know that sometimes, you just have to let some of them drop.

Some things are more important than others. We have to determine what our priorities are when it comes to raising our children. We need to determine the right balls to allow to fall to the ground. You may have to choose not to make the bed every day. You may have to turn off the TV for a long time. You may not be able to spend much time socializing on Facebook. You might see more loads of laundry lying around than you would like. The fact is, you can't do it all without sacrificing some crucial lifestyle habits as a family. And because you picked up this book, you know that healthy lifestyle habits is something you need to work on. You can't afford to sacrifice that any longer.

The amount of attention and care you invest in shaping your children's nutritional and fitness choices charts the course for the rest of their lives. It really *is* a big deal.

Sometimes, Love Means Saying No

We love our children and would do anything for them. If we knew we were harming them in some way—perhaps by being lax in monitoring their health habits—wouldn't we want to stop and start doing the right things?

I like what Jesus says about the nature of parents to give good things to their children: "If your children ask for a fish, do you give them a snake instead? Or if they ask for an egg, do you give them a scorpion? Of course not!" (Luke 11:11-12 NLT). The problem, however, is that our kids often ask for stuff that's not good for them (like fast food). And we think we show them love when we give in and say yes.

But then what happens? When we allow our kids to be in charge of our decision-making, they become the boss. They take over our job. They become the parent. Obviously, a family won't function well when children are running the house!

I know there are daily battles you fight with your kids. The trick is to pick your battles wisely. I want to challenge you to pick the battle of good health. This is a fight where you need to quit raising the white flag. You need to fight for the health of your children because this war really is a matter of life or death.

From the time our children are born, we try to give them the very best we can. We buy the best baby food and take them to the doctor any time they have the tiniest sniffle. We move to homes in the best school districts and sign them up for activities that we hope will grow them in some way, whether athletically or intellectually. We focus on doing all these things and more so that they have the best shot at a good life. In this hustle and bustle, sometimes we forget that the foundation of success is good health.

As parents, we have the power to ensure that our children do not fall prey to all the bad stuff that can result from being overweight and possibly even obese. These include conditions, illnesses, and diseases that can cripple them as they become adults. I want to talk about a few of them.

Silent Destroyers

According to the Mayo Clinic's website, childhood obesity puts children on the path to diabetes, high blood pressure, and high cholesterol. These are health problems that only adults used to suffer from. If you don't pay attention to your child's health now, you are essentially creating a breeding ground for these health issues as they get older.

Type 2 diabetes is an obesity-related illness that has drastically increased in children and teens. Diabetes is a condition in which a person has high blood sugar because the body can't make enough or can't properly use insulin. In order for your body to function optimally, your blood-sugar levels need to be in a particular target range. When the body isn't producing enough insulin or the body isn't processing it properly, this healthy range gets out of whack.

It's tough to detect type 2 diabetes in children because many symptoms may be mild or nonexistent. A blood test is required to properly diagnose this disease. According to the Centers for Disease Control and Prevention (CDC), children who have type 2 diabetes are generally between 10 and 19 years old, obese, and have a strong family history of type 2 diabetes.

This surge of diabetes in children and teens is attributed to lifestyle choices that lead to poor health. These include eating foods high in fat and calories (such as fast food), eating too much sugar (such as soda and candy), eating larger portions, and not getting enough exercise.

High blood pressure is another health condition that can result from being overweight. It affects only 3 percent of children and teens, according to the American Heart Association's website. This may seem like a small number, but it has risen over the years and is attributed to a poor diet, excess weight, and an insufficient amount of physical activity. High blood pressure is a really big deal because if left untreated, it can lead to damage of the kidneys, brain, heart, and eyes.

Blood pressure is the force of the blood pushing against the artery walls. When a person has high blood pressure, there is a higher than normal pressure inside the arteries, and the heart has a harder time pumping blood throughout the body. When the heart has to work harder than it needs to, it puts stress on your heart and makes it more difficult to get the necessary blood to your vital organs.

High cholesterol is another health problem on the rise. High cholesterol is something we need to pay attention to because it can create a material called plaque that builds up on the walls of the arteries. Plaque can prohibit the blood from flowing through the arteries and can even cause a heart attack and stroke if left untreated.

Three factors cause high cholesterol levels in children—heredity, diet, and obesity (notice the trend?). Most children with high cholesterol have a parent with high cholesterol. If this condition runs in your family, get your child diagnosed if you suspect they might suffer from the illness. It's easy to find out if this is the case. Just ask your pediatrician for a simple blood test. It's also fairly simple to treat high cholesterol. You have to put your child on a healthy diet (basically eating natural foods that are low in fat and good for you) and an exercise program. Medication might be in order for severe cases.

More than Feeling Blue

Another side effect of childhood weight problems and obesity is low self-esteem and depression. Being overweight impacts not only a child's physical body, it also impacts their emotional and mental states.

Childhood should be a time free of anxiety. It shouldn't be a time when your child is worried and depressed about his weight. If you were an overweight child, as I was, you know how painful that experience can be.

There are many things we can't control about our children, but one thing we can do something about is their weight. No one wants their child to be the last kid on the team picked to play kickball or an object of ridicule because of her size. No one wants their child to feel less-than or like a loser.

Our middle son, Pearson, was about 20 pounds overweight when we came home from the ranch. He was always a little shy and self-conscious when it came to those extra pounds. He is the most sensitive of our three children, and it pained me to know how bad he felt about himself. As I saw him get healthier when he lost the weight, I also saw his self-esteem blossom. As a mother, this was such a rewarding thing to witness.

Unhealthy Building Blocks Lead to Unhealthy Adult Habits

There are several more reasons why we need to take the health of our children seriously. One main reason is that an overweight child is much more likely to be an overweight adult. One study found that approximately 80 percent of children who were overweight between the ages of 10–15 years were obese at age 25.[1] Another study reports that 25 percent of obese adults were overweight as children, and that if unhealthy weight gain starts before the age of 8, then obesity in adulthood is likely to be more severe.[2] The idea that "a little baby fat never hurt anyone" is not true. It can hurt your child for the rest of his or her life.

Here's something else to think about. Once your body creates a fat cell, it never gets rid of it. The fat cell can shrink as you lose weight, but it is always there available to be filled up. And fat cells generally are not created in a person's body after puberty; the one exception is if an adult gains a considerable amount of weight. But for the most part, the number of fat cells a person has is determined in childhood. When kids become overweight, they create more fat cells than they would if they were at a healthy weight.

Fat cells also have memory. Once they have been full, they want to be full again. This is why once someone has been overweight, it becomes much more difficult for him to stay slim later in life. This is why it is so vital that we help our children get and stay healthy. We don't want them entering adulthood with the propensity to store fat, be obese, and be generally unhealthy. We don't want to create a disadvantage for them so early on.

Here's another sobering fact. Childhood obesity more than doubles the risk of dying before age 55, according to a study published in the *New England Journal of Medicine* and conducted by Dr. William C. Knowler, chief of the Diabetes Epidemiology and Clinical Research Section of the National Institute of Diabetes and Digestive and Kidney Diseases.

More Facts

The list of the dangers of childhood obesity is ever-growing. Extra weight on your child's body can cause lung problems, leading to ailments such as asthma. Sleep apnea (a condition where your child has abnormal breathing patterns while sleeping) can be a complication of childhood obesity. Being obese can create hormone imbalances for your child that can cause puberty to start earlier than expected.

Extra weight can even affect the way your kid's feet are formed. Did you know that flattened arches are often developed during childhood? An article in the June 21, 2010 edition of *USA Today* states that extra pounds can take a toll on feet, causing conditions such as flat feet, inflamed tendons, and sore feet. A spokesman for the American College of Foot and Ankle Surgeons said, "The foot was made to carry the average body, of maybe up to 200 pounds. When you add 100 or 200 pounds, it overloads the tendons, the ligaments, and the bones." While your child may not be 100 pounds overweight, any excess weight puts undue pressure on their feet. Likewise, Dr. Wendy J. Pomerantz of Cincinnati Children's Hospital Medical Center found obese children had more leg, ankle, and foot injuries than normal-weight children.[3]

Body Mass Index Table

Height (inches)	Normal						Overweight					Obese										Extreme Obesity															
BMI	19	20	21	22	23	24	25	26	27	28	29	30	31	32	33	34	35	36	37	38	39	40	41	42	43	44	45	46	47	48	49	50	51	52	53	54
												Body Weight (pounds)																								
58	91	96	100	105	110	115	119	124	129	134	138	143	148	153	158	162	167	172	177	181	186	191	196	201	205	210	215	220	224	229	234	239	244	248	253	258
59	94	99	104	109	114	119	124	128	133	138	143	148	153	158	163	168	173	178	183	188	193	198	203	208	212	217	222	227	232	237	242	247	252	257	262	267
60	97	102	107	112	118	123	128	133	138	143	148	153	158	163	168	174	179	184	189	194	199	204	209	215	220	225	230	235	240	245	250	255	261	266	271	276
61	100	106	111	116	122	127	132	137	143	148	153	158	164	169	174	180	185	190	195	201	206	211	217	222	227	232	238	243	248	254	259	264	269	275	280	285
62	104	109	115	120	126	131	136	142	147	153	158	164	169	175	180	186	191	196	202	207	213	218	224	229	235	240	246	251	256	262	267	273	278	284	289	295
63	107	113	118	124	130	135	141	146	152	158	163	169	175	180	186	191	197	203	208	214	220	225	231	237	242	248	254	259	265	270	276	282	287	293	299	304
64	110	116	122	128	134	140	145	151	157	163	169	174	180	186	192	197	204	209	215	221	227	232	238	244	250	256	262	267	273	279	285	291	296	302	308	314
65	114	120	126	132	138	144	150	156	162	168	174	180	186	192	198	204	210	216	222	228	234	240	246	252	258	264	270	276	282	288	294	300	306	312	318	324
66	118	124	130	136	142	148	155	161	167	173	179	186	192	198	204	210	216	223	229	235	241	247	253	260	266	272	278	284	291	297	303	309	315	322	328	334
67	121	127	134	140	146	153	159	166	172	178	185	191	198	204	211	217	223	230	236	242	249	255	261	268	274	280	287	293	299	306	312	319	325	331	338	344
68	125	131	138	144	151	158	164	171	177	184	190	197	203	210	216	223	230	236	243	249	256	262	269	276	282	289	295	302	308	315	322	328	335	341	348	354
69	128	135	142	149	155	162	169	176	182	189	196	203	209	216	223	230	236	243	250	257	263	270	277	284	291	297	304	311	318	324	331	338	345	351	358	365
70	132	139	146	153	160	167	174	181	188	195	202	209	216	222	229	236	243	250	257	264	271	278	285	292	299	306	313	320	327	334	341	348	355	362	369	376
71	136	143	150	157	165	172	179	186	193	200	208	215	222	229	236	243	250	257	265	272	279	286	293	301	308	315	322	329	338	343	351	358	365	372	379	386
72	140	147	154	162	169	177	184	191	199	206	213	221	228	235	242	250	258	265	272	279	287	294	302	309	316	324	331	338	346	353	361	368	375	383	390	397
73	144	151	159	166	174	182	189	197	204	212	219	227	235	242	250	257	265	272	280	288	295	302	310	318	325	333	340	348	355	363	371	378	386	393	401	408
74	148	155	163	171	179	186	194	202	210	218	225	233	241	249	256	264	272	280	287	295	303	311	319	326	334	342	350	358	365	373	381	389	396	404	412	420
75	152	160	168	176	184	192	200	208	216	224	232	240	248	256	264	272	279	287	295	303	311	319	327	335	343	351	359	367	375	383	391	399	407	415	423	431
76	156	164	172	180	189	197	205	213	221	230	238	246	254	263	271	279	287	295	304	312	320	328	336	344	353	361	369	377	385	394	402	410	418	426	435	443

Source: Adapted from Clinical Guidelines on the Identification, Evaluation, and Treatment of Overweight and Obesity in Adults: The Evidence Report.

When we say that obesity can affect you from the top of your head to the soles of your feet, we're not kidding.

Is My Child Part of This Problem?

Is your child at risk of being overweight or even obese? How can you tell? Phillip and I like to evaluate healthy weight by using the Body Mass Index (BMI) chart.

BMI is a number calculated from a person's weight and height that is a reliable indicator of whether your child is overweight. It's not foolproof, however, because it doesn't take into consideration how much muscle a child has. Muscle weighs more than fat, and some kids naturally have more muscle than others. Also, the BMI chart can be a little skewed during periods of rapid growth. Still, it's a generally solid guideline to use. The best way to get an accurate reading is to get a scale that measures body fat, weight, and hydration levels or make an appointment with your child's doctor.

If you decide to calculate your child's BMI on your own, you first need to take some measurements. Measure your child's height and write it down. Then weigh your child and write that number down. Compare these numbers with the chart on the previous page or insert them into the handy BMI calculator on the Centers for Disease Control website (http://apps.nccd.cdc.gov/dnpabmi/).

If you find that your child falls in the overweight or obese range, don't waste time beating yourself up about it or blaming your poor parental skills. The key is to realize that starting today, you can change this number. You can change the way your family eats. You can change the way your family exercises (or doesn't at all). You can even change your child's health if she is suffering from weight-related conditions. You can make a difference.

Reading this book and working through the 90 challenges in Part 2 is a great first step. Make this a priority and read the challenges together as a family at the breakfast or dinner table, right before or after you help your children with their homework, or the first thing when they come home from school. Make these challenges a part of your routine to help your children understand that you are on their side and you want to help them be healthy.

Don't judge or make your kids feel bad if they are overweight. Support them and let them know this is something you can conquer together. When I was a little girl, my grandmother would make negative comments about my weight all the time. She meant well, but it made me feel as if she didn't approve of (or even like) me. Your child needs to know that you love her and support her in every area, including her journey to become healthy.

How to Make Change

As you read this chapter, you may have noticed a continual theme. Like a drumbeat, the words *healthy eating* and *exercise* sound over and over. Many life-threatening conditions can be prevented by making changes in our diet and in our level of activity. Why do we not do it? I believe three culprits prevent us from making these changes—time management, energy, and motivation.

We must take inventory of our time. You may think that you already have every single second scheduled to a tee and you have absolutely no extra time, but I bet you can adjust your schedule and incorporate small changes that will give you more time to spend on your health. You can cook food ahead of time so you always have a snack on hand to avoid the drive-thru window. Instead of throwing bags of chips or cookies in your children's lunch box, pack a piece of fruit. Do homework with your child at the park, so after he or she is finished, you can run around and play together and squeeze in some physical activity. See what I mean? Making little changes in your routine can make a big difference.

What about energy? Many parents I know complain of not having enough energy to make health a priority. They are simply too tired. This is where you have to make sure that you are taking care of your health first so that you can help your family. (This is also the best way to role model healthy habits for your children. If you don't do it, why should they?)

When you make time for exercise, you actually have more energy than when you are sedentary. I know this is true from personal experience. If I start my morning with exercise, I have tons of energy for the rest of my day. I turn into the Energizer Bunny. I just keep going and going and going.

Finally, sometimes we don't make changes because we don't have the motivation to change. But what is more motivational than our children? Our kids should be the biggest motivators in creating a healthy lifestyle at home. I don't know of anything that can move me more than when I know my child has a need. I like to think one thing most parents have in common is a desire to see their children live long, healthy lives. And I believe you, as a parent, will do anything to give them a foundation for a great quality of life. So make the commitment to make change. Let them be your motivation to eat better and start moving more. We will be with you every step of the way!

How Healthy Are Your Kids?

Let's find out how healthy your kids are. The quiz below is a great starting point for you as a parent to know what kind of commitment you will need to make to get the change-ball rolling. Circle your answers and tally your score.

1. My kids eat fast food...
   a) once a week (2)
   b) at least five times a week (3)
   c) once or twice a month as a special treat (1)
   d) every day (4)

2. When we do something together as a family, we like to...
   a) go out to eat (4)
   b) go to the movies (3)
   c) do something active such as play sports or go hiking (1)
   d) go to an amusement park (2)

3. The drink that my kids have most with meals is...
   a) soda (4)
   b) water (1)
   c) milk (2)
   d) juice (3)

4. My kids watch TV and play on the computer or video games...
   a) an hour a day (2)
   b) two hours a day (3)
   c) three or more hours a day (4)
   d) less than an hour a day (1)

5. My kids participate in regular exercise...

    a) 30 minutes a day, five days a week (1)

    b) an hour a day, three days a week (2)

    c) once a week (if we're lucky) (3)

    d) never (4)

6. We eat dinner together as a family...

    a) during major holidays (4)

    b) once a week (2)

    c) at least five days a week (1)

    d) on weekends when we go to a sit-down restaurant (3)

If you scored:

6 to 12 points—Green light! All systems are go. You are traveling in the right direction as a family. As you read this book you will continue to learn more about great health.

13 to 18 points—Yellow light! Caution. On the way to trouble ahead. You can find your way to the path toward great health by reading how you can create a healthy family environment.

18 to 24 points—Red alert! You need to get your family in the "Challenge" ASAP! Don't worry. Today can be the first day of your family's journey toward a life of good health.

Whatever your score, in the following chapters we will equip you to make your family life not just happy but healthy. Whether it's learning about the best foods to fuel your body or discovering creative ways of exercising as a family, the time to challenge yourself to be a healthy family is now. And the best place to start...is with you!

3

Your Kids Are Watching You

—————————— A Word from Amy ——————————

I'm sure most of you are familiar with the saying, "Do what I say and not what I do." I've found that far too many parents have this mentality when they're instructing or guiding their kids. And it's usually when they're trying to get their children to do something that they're not willing to do themselves.

We warn our kids not to smoke, though we smoke two packs of cigarettes a day. We demand they get good grades, though we are slacking in our job. We preach the dangers of alcohol, though we make sure to keep a six-pack of beer in the fridge. We scold them for drinking too much soda, yet we have a stash of cookies hidden in the back of the cupboard. We encourage them to play outside as we sit on the couch watching *Oprah* and clutching the remote to our ever-growing belly.

We give good advice to our children and warn them of potential danger because we know it's for their benefit. It's not as though we're sending them a wrong message, at least not verbally. But if we don't back our words with our actions, our well-intentioned suggestions are meaningless.

Set the Example

It seems that sometimes we expect more of our children than we expect of ourselves. We hold them to a high standard, but we have no bar of expectations of our own. I've preached countless messages to my kids that I have been unable to reinforce with my behaviors. But I've learned something in that process. You can't expect your children to do things you are not willing to do. You have to set an example for them to follow. You have to be the leader who paves the way if you want them to make the right choices.

Many years ago I taught a program for three year olds at my church. During the training class, the director said something I'll never forget: "Children will always rise to the level that you expect of them." In other words, if you establish boundaries and rules and expect your children to follow them, they will rise to that level.

But let's be honest. How can we establish boundaries, rules, and standards that we are not willing to follow ourselves? It's like a police officer who has a record of drinking and driving arresting someone for a DUI. We can't set expectations for our children and believe they will rise to those expectations if we are hypocrites. It simply won't work. We need to look in the mirror and realize that change in our family starts with us. No more excuses. If we want our children to change, we have to change too.

I applaud you if you are setting a good example for your children. You've won half the battle in raising them up to where you want them to go. The Bible says, "Train up a child in the way he should go, and when he is old he will not turn from it" (Proverbs 22:6). This verse speaks volumes.

What do you think is the best training for your kids? Not just telling them what to do, but "training" them. You are living by example. You are showing them the ropes. You are teaching them how it's done through doing the right things yourself.

When I was a little girl, my mother had a plaque on her wall that depicted a beautiful poem, "Children Learn What They Live" by Dorothy Law Nolte. It talked about how children will learn unhealthy and damaging behaviors from their parents. If their mom or dad exhibits anger, the child will learn how to be mad. If the parent is critical, the child will learn how to condemn. Likewise, if the parent is positive, the child will learn how to maintain a good attitude. If the parent is supportive, the child will learn how to be confident. Whatever attitudes and behaviors characterize the parents will be reflected in their child.

I like this poem because it reminds me that our children will be influenced by the environment we surround them with. What we do matters more than what we say. Think about your home environment. What do you project in your actions and behaviors that your child might emulate or be affected by? Good things? Or not-so-good things?

In this journey to transform your life and live your dreams of being healthier, happier, and more fit, inspire your family by leading by example.

Make the right choices. Do the right things. And watch how your family will notice and start to emulate your healthy habits.

Ignite Passion

Have you ever met a family that had such a strong passion about a particular activity that it almost defined who they were as a family? Know any families who are college football fanatics, for instance? Come football season, they decorate their cars with stickers sporting their team's logo, they wear their team's jersey, they paint their faces with their team's colors on game day, they schedule their life around game days, and you can find them tailgating at every home game.

The kids who are raised in this type of family weren't born with such a huge passion for football. It was created in them by watching how excited their parents got when football season rolled around. It was created in them by being enveloped in the hype. Somewhere along the line, football madness became a normal part of these kids' family life. They are the football family. It's just what they do.

I know so many families who share similar passions. I know a family who is really into building houses for the homeless. Another family I know loves camping. You can be passionate about almost anything.

I think the best thing to throw your passion into as a family is health and fitness. You can make eating right and exercising a part of your family identity so it becomes synonymous with who you are.

Over the last several years, I've had the privilege of running in and hosting several races. I'm always excited to see mothers and fathers running with jogging strollers or running with their older kids at their side. These parents are role modeling a healthy lifestyle for their children and igniting a passion for an activity their children will likely engage in as they get older. These families run. It's what they do.

Being healthy can be something you and your children just do. Ignite the passion and set the pace. You won't be disappointed.

Simple Steps

By now, most of you understand that establishing good health and fitness habits in the home begins with you. But exactly how do you do this? What are some starting points? This book answers those questions in the next chapters, but here are a few simple steps you can take to lead your family in the direction of a better you. Most experts in the health and medical fields suggest that doing these things will help build a healthy lifestyle.

Eat a healthy, well-balanced diet. By maintaining a healthy diet, you decrease your risk of obesity, diabetes, hypertension, heart disease, and some cancers. This fact is supported by studies from the American Heart Association, Centers for Disease Control, American Diabetes Association, and American Cancer Society. All of these agencies agree that a healthy diet is the key to preventing life-threatening diseases.

We'll talk about this more in chapter 4, but here is a main key to good nutrition: eat more natural foods and fewer processed foods. Stick with fruits, vegetables, whole grains, and lean meats. Don't keep packaged or junk food in the house. If you have unhealthy food or snacks around, you and your kids will be more likely to eat them. We have a bowl right on the kitchen counter that is always full of all kinds of fruits. We also store in the fridge little baggies of veggies (such as baby carrots) that are quick and delicious to snack on.

Exercise regularly. According to the American Heart Association and the American Diabetes Association, exercise also helps decrease the risk of obesity, heart disease, diabetes, and hypertension. Not only that, but it helps boost your immune system. It reduces stress. It helps keep the blood circulating through your heart and lungs, which gives you more energy. Exercise even makes you sleep better.

By exercising regularly, you are not only improving your health and happiness, you are also teaching your children they need to be active. Being active with your kids is a great way to be healthy and an opportunity to spend quality time together. Play a round of tennis. Take them hiking. Go for a walk. Play Frisbee in the park. Go swimming at the local pool. They will soon develop a love for fitness and will appreciate the time you spend with them. Our family loves to go for a walk around the neighborhood after dinner. It gives us a chance to stretch our legs and catch up on the day's happenings.

Spend less time watching television. By turning off the TV, you and your child will have more time to do other things together. Instead of staring at a screen watching other people live their lives, you can learn a new hobby, play a sport, read together, or go old-school and simply get out in the fresh air and play. (We'll talk more about the dangers of watching too much TV in chapter 5.)

An article in *Science Daily*[4] connects childhood obesity with watching too much television. It offers the American Academy of Pediatrics (AAP) suggestion that children watch no more than two hours of television a day. Also, an article found on www.kidshealth.org (September 2010) indicates that spending time with your children each day makes them more likely to make healthy choices.

Television, computer, video games, iPods, Nintendo DS—all this new technology meant to entertain our children is causing more harm than good. Unplug these devices. Take the batteries out. Participate in activities as a family that stimulate the mind (such as reading, board games, going to a museum, or visiting an art gallery) and—try this on for size—engage in good old-fashioned communication.

And remember, don't just limit your children's TV or video game time, limit your TV time as well. Instead of watching your favorite reality show or HBO drama, go for a walk or take your child to the bookstore or the playground.

If you choose to drink alcohol, drink responsibly. If you don't drink, great. If you do, make the choice to limit your alcohol intake. According to the Centers for Disease Control[5], alcohol is a factor in 41 percent of all deaths in the United States from motor vehicle accidents. Excessive alcohol consumption is associated with approximately 75,000 deaths per year.

I know we can't make our kids not drink when they get older, but we can set the foundation to prevent underage drinking. Don't drink and drive. Don't use alcohol to fill a void in your life or to numb yourself from pain. Model the right behavior in front of your kids and show them the dangers of alcohol. Phillip and I live by the principle that anything in excess is not good (this includes drinking alcohol), and we make sure we communicate this to our kids by example.

Don't smoke or use any tobacco products. This is an easy one. The American Legacy Foundation reports that children of smokers are twice as likely as kids from nonsmoking homes to try a cigarette or smoke regularly. Extensive research has been conducted on the dangers of cigarette smoking. Smoking can cause asthma, lung disease, and even lung cancer. Smoking also has hazardous secondhand effects.

If you smoke, now is the time to quit and show your family that you are motivated to improve yourself even if it's hard work. Don't be a prisoner of cigarettes or tobacco. It doesn't affect just your health; it affects the health of your children as well.

Read. Reading is a favorite hobby in the Parham household. Our children have grown up watching Phillip and me cuddle up with a good book at the end of the day. This has developed in them a love for reading. The American Literacy Association tells us that reading is the foundation of learning and knowledge. I found that reading is a great way for me to relax and unwind after a long, hard day. It's certainly better than eating ice cream, downing a glass of wine, smoking a cigarette, or watching TV.

Life is stressful for most of us, and we need to build in a designated time for relaxation. This is also a great way to create and reinforce bonds with your children. I love to spend a rainy day indoors with my kids and read a book together. It's a great feeling.

Wear a seat belt. When my children were little, we had a ritual before we started the car. We had a checklist that Phillip and I went through and our kids responded in unison. It went something like this: "Snacks? Check! Sunglasses? Check! Mirrors adjusted? Check! Veggie Tales CD? Check! Seat belts on? Check!" The last check was always the loudest one.

Putting on your seat belt is such a simple thing, but many parents still forget to do it. To this day my kids still police me about "clicking in," and they always make sure to click in themselves. Model safe behavior for your children. Wear your seat belt.

Deal with stress appropriately. This is a tough suggestion for any parent, but think about this: Children learn how to cope by watching their parents deal with stressful situations. Stress usually comes from life changes such as getting a new job, moving to a new town, dealing with illness, and switching schools. Most people don't like change, even if it's good for them. The kind of change is not as important as our reaction to it. Your reaction will determine the outcome of your situation.

Even when you don't think your children are watching you, know that they are. And they are also learning from your behaviors. If you yell and scream when you're upset, they'll learn to do the same. If you are even-tempered and levelheaded, they will react in similar fashion. When conflict arises, teach your children to discuss things calmly and rationally. Exhibit calm and rational behavior such as patiently listening to all sides of an argument and showing respect for all parties involved. One thing is certain: stressful times will come. It's up to you to handle them the best way possible.

Maintain close relationships with your spouse, family, and friends. Being socially well-rounded is critical to leading a balanced life. While it's necessary to spend quality time with your children, you should also spend time with other people you are close to, such as your spouse, your sister, or your best friend. This teaches your children that healthy and nurturing relationships are a big deal. They help us grow and develop and give us an opportunity to practice love, mercy, and kindness. I like what Anthony Robbins said, "The quality of your life is the quality of your relationships."

Phillip and I have regular date nights without the kids. We don't do this because we don't enjoy or want to be around our kids. We do this to cultivate our relationship so we can become a better wife and a better husband. In turn, we become better parents. Our children appreciate that Phillip and I want to spend time together as a couple. They really get a kick out of it.

We also invest in our friendships. Our world does not revolve solely around our family or our problems. As human beings, we all need each other.

Make a difference in the lives of others. It is our God-given responsibility to help others who are less fortunate than we are. The Bible says,

> What good is it, my brothers, if a man claims to have faith but has no deeds? Can such faith save him? Suppose a brother or sister is without clothes and daily food. If one of you says to him, "Go, I wish you well; keep warm and well fed," but does nothing about his physical needs, what good is it? In the same way, faith by itself, if it is not accompanied by action, is dead (James 2:14-17).

If you are a believer, you have a responsibility to help those in need. This is an act of faith that takes our belief beyond words and creeds. It moves us toward action. God made us to take care of others. I've found this to be a cyclic thing. When you start doing good to others, you'll notice others start doing good to you. When you help out someone, you'll find help just when you need it.

Teach your kids this cardinal lesson. Set the example for them. Do something that, as the movie title says, pays it forward. It can be as simple as picking up trash at your local park, volunteering at a charitable organization, or helping a neighbor mow her yard.

Most of us have been blessed beyond measure. God is pleased when we are faithful stewards of what we have. Teach your children to be generous, charitable, and aware of others. They will likely keep those same characteristics as adults and therefore live a more meaningful and enriching life. There is no greater gift than to help someone who is less fortunate than we are. The rewards far surpass anything tangible or material.

One Step at a Time

These are just a few areas in which you can be a role model. Don't get overwhelmed if you feel as if this list means you have to turn your life upside down. Take one recommendation at a time and focus on making the right adjustments in that area. You could start by shutting off the TV every now and then or throwing out all the junk food in your house. Once you think you have overcome an area, start working on another. If you find you are dealing with something that's too hard to change on your own, get outside help. Find a therapist or support group to help you.

We can no longer simply wish for change in our families; we have to initiate that change. I'm not saying it's going to be easy. It's like John Porter said, "People underestimate their capacity for change. There is never a right time to do a difficult thing. A leader's job is to help people have vision of their potential." Your job as a mother or father is to lead your children by example. Show them what is possible for them. Help them see the vision of a healthy and fit lifestyle.

When God gave you your children, He entrusted you to take care of them to the best of your knowledge and ability. When you set a good example for your children, you are actually honoring and serving God in your actions. Trust Him to give you the strength to make the changes necessary to make your family the best it can be.

How Healthy Are You?

Here is a simple assessment to gauge the quality of your health. I recommend talking with your family doctor to determine if you are at a healthy weight and what, if any, medical problems you may have as a result of any excess weight.

Read these questions and review your answers (with a doctor if possible). Identify some areas that you may need to change or improve.

1. What is your blood pressure? _____. You can have your blood pressure checked by your doctor or visit a local pharmacy that offers self-service blood pressure stations. Compare your number to the chart below. Is it in a healthy range?

Category	Blood Pressure
Normal	<120/80
Prehypertension	120–139/80–89
Hypertension: Stage 1	140–159/90–99
Hypertension: Stage 2	160–179/100–109 ≥180/110

National Institutes of Health, August 2004

2. How much do you weigh? _____. Most of you have a scale at home or can get weighed at your doctor's office. Compare your number with the chart on the next page. Is it in a healthy range? To calculate your frame type, place your thumb and index finger around your wrist. If your finger overlaps the thumb, you are "Small Frame." If they touch, you are "Medium Frame." If they do not touch, you are "Large Frame."

3. What is your body mass index (BMI)? _____. We talked about this in the previous chapter. The Department of Health and Human Services has a nifty BMI calculator that's easy to use (www.nhlbisupport.com/bmi/). Just plug in your height and weight and it will figure it out for you. This site will also tell you if you have a healthy BMI.

4. Do you drink at least eight glasses of water a day? If not, you're not drinking enough water. Do you drink soda or other sugary drinks instead?

Height and Weight Table for Women			
Height Feet Inches	Small Frame	Medium Frame	Large Frame
4' 10"	102–111	109–121	118–131
4' 11"	103–113	111–123	120–134
5' 0"	104–115	113–126	122–137
5' 1"	106–118	115–129	125–140
5' 2"	108–121	118–132	128–143
5' 3"	111–124	121–135	131–147
5' 4"	114–127	124–138	134–151
5' 5"	117–130	127–141	137–155
5' 6"	120–133	130–144	140–159
5' 7"	123–136	133–147	143–163
5' 8"	126–139	136–150	146–167
5' 9"	129–142	139–153	149–170
5' 10"	132–145	142–156	152–173
5' 11"	135–148	145–159	155–176
6' 0"	138–151	148–162	158–179

Height and Weight Table for Men			
Height Feet Inches	Small Frame	Medium Frame	Large Frame
5' 2"	128–134	131–141	138–150
5' 3"	130–136	133–143	140–153
5" 4"	132–138	135–145	142–156
5' 5"	134–140	137–148	144–160
5' 6"	136–142	139–151	146–164
5' 7"	138–145	142–154	149–168
5' 8"	140–148	145–157	152–172
5' 9"	142–151	148–160	155–176
5' 10"	144–154	151–163	158–180
5' 11"	146–157	154–166	161–184
6' 0"	149–160	157–170	164–188
6' 1"	152–164	160–174	168–192
6' 2"	155–168	164–178	172–197
6' 3"	158–172	167–182	176–202
6' 4"	162–176	171–187	181–207

5. How many hours do you spend watching TV, socializing online, or surfing the Internet? Be honest with yourself. Can you cut down on some of this time to engage in activities that are more active, healthy, and mentally stimulating?

Use your answers as a barometer to measure the kind of example you are setting for your children. If you need to improve some aspects of your lifestyle, I encourage you to work on them during this "Challenge." Don't feel bad if your assessment isn't so great. Use it as a learning tool to start developing better health habits.

Plan of Action

- Set the example. Role-model good health for your children.

- Be passionate about a particular healthy activity or a general healthy lifestyle. Get excited about it so your kids will catch your enthusiasm.

- Talk to a physician or evaluate your own health to determine what areas you can improve.

- Take small steps to increase the quality of your health each day. Believe me, your kids will notice.

We've got a lot of learning to do when it comes to what we put in our mouth. In the next chapter, you'll learn how to eat, what to eat, when to eat, and the best and worst foods for you and your family. Don't worry. Eating healthy is not boring or tasteless. We're going to make this as delicious for you as we can.

4

Nutrition Sense for Your Family

I wish my parents had taught me about good nutrition. Though my mother put plenty of vegetables on the table, we weren't given any guidance about what food was good for us and why. I ate what I liked, and my parents reinforced that behavior. If it tasted good, I ate it. If I ate it, they bought it.

As a parent, it's crucial to know the building blocks of good nutrition so you can teach your kids how and what to eat. Good nutrition is not a diet; it's a lifestyle. Proper eating habits and lifestyle modification are things you can learn to do that have lasting benefits.

The starting point is to understand why we eat. We eat to fuel our bodies. We don't eat to comfort our emotions, to make us feel better, to fill a void, or to satisfy our cravings. We eat to give our body the fuel it needs to work at an optimal level. I like to say that we eat to live. Every time you sit down to eat a meal or snack, you have to ask yourself whether it will fuel your body or slow it down. This is a mind game you have to conquer and this is something you must teach your kids. If they learn early enough that food is not an emotional crutch, they will be more likely to live by this lifestyle principle as they get older.

Having a nutritious lifestyle doesn't mean you can't ever have some ice cream or a piece of cake. The key is moderation. A slice of pizza every now and then won't compromise your health; just don't make it a habit. We've also learned that when you snack or treat on something, there are also healthier alternatives. We'll talk about some of this later in this chapter.

The Big Picture

Think Natural

Good nutrition means choosing foods that are natural, such as fresh

47

fruits, vegetables, nuts, and lean meats. Natural means that the food is as close to its original state as possible and has not been or is only minimally processed. Your body functions best when it is nourished by natural foods.

Did you know that our bodies are efficient at healing themselves with the right foods? You'll notice the more natural you eat, the less you are sick. Americans are among the sickest people in the world. I believe it comes back to our diet. Too many people in our country eat at fast-food restaurants too often. All that preservative-filled junk is what is sending us to an early grave. It's this simple: Stop eating fast food. Drive past the drive-thru.

Below is a list of basic foods that has helped Amy and me keep the weight off. We feed our children from the basic sources of food below (the breakdown of protein, carbohydrates, and fat will be explained later in this chapter). This preliminary list will also give you an idea of what we mean by eating natural. A more comprehensive shopping list will be discussed in chapter 7 and listed in appendix A.

Protein Source

- eat only lean cuts of meat: chicken, turkey, fish, beef (sirloin or round cuts), lamb
- turkey (sausage, ground, whole)
- eggs
- vegetarian choices include firm tofu, tempeh, cooked lentils, kidney beans, lima beans, black beans, chickpeas

Carb Sources

- oatmeal (not instant)
- fruit
- vegetables, vegetables, vegetables
- brown rice
- whole grains

Fat Sources

- olive oil (the best to use for cooking; use cold-pressed, extra virgin olive oil)

- safflower oil
- coconut oil (great for high-heat cooking)
- almond oil
- avocado

How Much Should We Eat?

There is so much different information about how much and what kids need to eat at a particular age. According to the U.S. Department of Agriculture's new Food Pyramid, the five main food groups that your child's meals and snacks should come from are:

- Grains—any food made from wheat, rice, oats, cornmeal, barley, or another cereal grain. Eat whole grains such as whole-wheat bread, brown rice, and oatmeal.

- Vegetables—any vegetable or 100-percent vegetable juice.

- Fruits—any fruit or 100-percent fruit juice.

- Milk—all fluid milk products and many foods made from milk, such as cheese and butter.

- Meat and Beans—all foods made from meat, poultry, fish, dry beans or peas, eggs, nuts, and seeds are considered part of this group.

The chart on the following two pages specifies the amounts your child will need at different ages to maintain a healthy diet. Keep in mind this recommendation is based on children who get less than 30 minutes per day of moderate physical activity, beyond normal daily activities. Kids who are more physically active may be able to eat more.

(To get a better grasp on how much you need to eat as an adult, refer to our first book, *The 90-Day Fitness Challenge*, for more information.)

GRAINS

	Daily Recommendation	Daily Minimum Amount of Whole Grains
Children 2–3 years old	3-ounce equivalents	1½-ounce equivalents
Children 4–8 years old	4–5-ounce equivalents	2–2½-ounce equivalents
Girls 9–13 years old	5-ounce equivalents	3-ounce equivalents
Girls 14–18 years old	6-ounce equivalents	3-ounce equivalents
Boys 9–13 years old	6-ounce equivalents	3-ounce equivalents
Boys 14–18 years old	7-ounce equivalents	3½-ounce equivalents

VEGETABLES

	Daily Recommendation
Children 2–3 years old	1 cup
Children 4–8 years old	1½ cups
Girls 9–13 years old	2 cups
Girls 14–18 years old	2½ cups
Boys 9–13 years old	2½ cups
Boys 14–18 years old	3 cups

FRUITS

	Daily Recommendation
Children 2–3 years old	1 cup
Children 4–8 years old	1 to 1½ cups
Girls 9–13 years old	1½ cups
Girls 14–18 years old	1½ cups
Boys 9–13 years old	1½ cups
Boys 14–18 years old	2 cups

MILK

	Daily Recommendation
Children 2–3 years old	2 cups
Children 4–8 years old	2 cups
Girls 9–13 years old	3 cups
Girls 14–18 years old	3 cups
Boys 9–13 years old	3 cups
Boys 14–18 years old	3 cups

MEAT AND BEANS	
	Daily Recommendation
Children 2–3 years old	2-ounce equivalents
Children 4–8 years old	3–4-ounce equivalents
Girls 9–13 years old	5-ounce equivalents
Girls 14–18 years old	5-ounce equivalents
Boys 9–13 years old	5-ounce equivalents
Boys 14–18 years old	6-ounce equivalents

Tips for Success

Drink Your Water

Water is a vital component of good health because much of our bodies consist of it. If we don't drink enough, we become dehydrated and can get a whole slew of health problems. Here are a few of the reasons you and your family should be drinking more water:

- Keeps your energy up
- Keeps your weight down
- Removes waste and eliminates toxins
- Helps carry nutrients and oxygen to cells
- Cushions joints
- Helps body absorb nutrients
- Hydrates skin and hair
- Regulates body temperature

How much water is enough? Adults need to drink half their body's weight in ounces of water each day. So if you weigh 200 pounds, you should be drinking 100 ounces of water. For children, there isn't any magic number. Most experts suggest 6–8 ounces of water and more than that if they are playing or exercising hard.

Drinking water is a challenge for many kids because they prefer soda or other sugary drinks instead. (We'll talk more about the dangers of soda later in this chapter.) When Amy and I got back from the ranch, we got rid of all the soda in the house; now the only beverages we regularly stock are water and milk. We occasionally allow some fruit drinks such as apple, orange, or grape, but we make sure the sugar content is low or that it is 100-percent juice (no added sugar). We often tell our kids to drink equal parts fruit juice and water to cut down on the sugar content.

When we eliminated soda from our house, our boys complained like you wouldn't believe. Amy and I jokingly refer to our "soda ban" as ripping off a Band-Aid. One day the soda was just not available to our kids, and they couldn't do a thing about it. It took several months for them to quit whining about not being able to drink soda, but finally they developed a taste for water. After a year, they started using such words as *dehydration* and saying they needed more water.

Bring on the Fiber

Fiber is a nutrient we don't often talk about but is wildly important to our bodies. Fiber refers to carbohydrates that cannot be digested. It's present in all plants that are eaten for food, including fruits, vegetables, grains, and legumes.

Fiber benefits us in several ways:

- Curbs overeating because it fills us up.
- Steadies blood-sugar levels.
- Slows down fat absorption.
- Reduces cholesterol.
- Promotes bowel regularity.

Keep in mind that not all fiber is the same. There are two types of fiber, soluble and insoluble, and they affect your body in different ways. Soluble fiber absorbs water in the intestine and slows the rate of glucose digestion and absorption in the bloodstream. Insoluble fiber adds bulk and softness to your stool and aids elimination.

The best sources of soluble fiber are:

- oat bran
- kidney beans
- lentils
- sweet potatoes
- oranges
- broccoli

- pears
- apples
- barley
- peas

The best sources of insoluble fiber are:

- wheat bran
- legumes
- skin of fruit
- seeds and nuts, such as sunflower seeds, soybean nuts, almonds

Most experts recommend that children and adults consume at least 20 grams of dietary fiber (a mix of the two types) per day from food, not supplements. Unfortunately, most Americans don't consume that much. Incorporating more fiber into your diet is not that hard to do. Remember, think natural. The more natural you eat, the more fiber you will get. So just say no to processed foods and say yes to natural foods!

Balance Macronutrients

The three major macronutrients are carbohydrates, proteins, and fat. Many fad diets teach you to take one of these three out to trick your body into losing weight. You have to realize that your body needs them all.

Protein is the building block of muscle. Carbohydrates give us energy and are our greatest source of fuel. Fat helps burn stored body fat, gives us energy, and surrounds and protects our tissue and vital organs. It also regulates our body temperature and hormone production. Fat is beneficial in appropriate quantities (not more than 25 percent from your daily calories); too much or too little can be harmful.

Our nutrition coach, Dr. Rick Katouff, gives us this formula for incorporating the correct balance of macronutrients into our daily diet. This is especially helpful when preparing meals:

- 40–55 percent carbohydrates
- 20–30 percent protein
- 20–30 percent fat

When Amy started balancing her meals this way, she stopped having sugar cravings in the middle of the night. I believe eating with this correct proportion aligned her hormones the right way. When you eat with this macronutrient balance, you will notice several things. You will have more energy, fewer mood swings, and fewer afternoon crashes. Your kids will notice the same thing. So focus on having snacks and meals that are properly balanced with good complex carbohydrates and lean protein with a small amount of healthy fat.

We also recommend eating four or five smaller meals throughout the day instead of three large meals. Eating small, healthy snacks and meals gets your metabolism moving, keeps your energy up, and keeps your hunger at bay. You never want to sit down to a meal when you are famished because you will tend to overeat.

Watch Your Portion Sizes

Let's face it. Our kids have a whole different worldview than ours. It's unfortunate, but today's society teaches that bigger is better. We supersize everything—cars, houses, and meals (especially meals!). In this super-sized life, our food portions have gotten way out of control. People are simply eating too much. When you eat more than you're supposed to, it takes a long time for your body to digest all that extra food. The key is to eat for one, not for two or three.

A little over 30 years ago, the typical plate size was around 9 inches. Today it has ballooned to around 12 inches. Because our cupboards and restaurant shelves are full of big plates, we tend to eat more. One of my favorite books on this subject is *The 9-inch "Diet": Exposing the Big Conspiracy in America* by Alex Bogusky and Chuck Porter. They explain how our portions have drastically increased over the years and what we can do about it. I suggest you read it.

Here's a challenge for you. Look in your cabinet and measure the dinner plates you're currently using. How big are they? Are you surprised?

You may have noticed too that restaurants have bloated portion sizes. Have you seen a pasta dish at your favorite eatery lately? You could feed three of your family members with one dish! If you want to eat the correct portion and save money (what a great combination!), the next time your family is at a restaurant, share your entrée with your spouse or your children. Or as soon as the meal comes, ask for a take-out box and save half your meal for lunch the next day.

Here's another piece of advice: read labels (I'll talk more about that next) to find out the size of a single serving of chips, cereal, ice cream, and so on. Then compare that amount with how much you are feeding your family. I suspect you'll notice a drastic difference.

To help our family stay within a single-portion limit, we keep measuring cups and a food scale within reach in the kitchen. These are great tools to educate you into what a single portion looks like. Because I have a tendency to overeat, I always watch my portions, so I rely on these kitchen gadgets a lot.

Read Labels

Most people do not read food labels, but those labels are your best source of information for how many calories are in a food, what the ingredients are, and how nutritious it is. There are six basic items you need to look for when reading a label:

> **Ingredients**—If the ingredients list includes words I can't pronounce or I know are not good for me (such as high-fructose corn syrup or added sugar), I don't buy it.
>
> **Serving size**—This helps me determine how much of a product I should eat.
>
> **Calories**—I always pay attention to the number of calories in a serving size. As a general rule of thumb:
>
> - 40 calories per serving is low in calories
> - 100 calories per serving is moderate in calories
> - 400 calories or more per serving is high in calories

These numbers will vary for children. Our suggestion is simply to stick with eating whole, natural foods and limit processed foods and junk food so your kids don't have to count calories.

> **Sugar**—We always choose foods that are low in sugar. Our family avoids eating anything with added sugar. (More on the dangers of sugar later.)
>
> **Sodium**—We choose only foods that are low in salt. (More on this topic later.)

Fiber—Choose high-fiber foods with at least three grams of fiber per serving.

The Trade Game

Substitution is the name of the game. Eating healthy doesn't mean you have to sacrifice taste. We eat a lot of different foods that our kids enjoy, such as healthy fried chicken, pizza, and burgers. The key is to substitute unhealthy ingredients with healthy ones. In appendix B, you'll find a list of the top ten recipes we regularly make that kids just love!

Below are some examples of how you can create a healthy meal plan for your family by replacing unhealthy ingredients with healthy ones.

Instead of This:	Try This:
White flour	Whole-wheat flour
Mayonnaise	Mustard
Ketchup	Salsa
Ice cream	Frozen yogurt
White rice	Brown rice
Regular pasta	Wheat or quinoa pasta
White bread	Wheat bread or wraps or Ezekiel bread
Ground beef	Ground turkey or chicken
Whole milk	Skim milk
Sour cream	Plain low-fat yogurt
White, creamy sauces (such as Alfredo)	Red, tomato sauces (such as marinara)
Salt	Herb seasonings such as pepper, Mrs. Dash, and others

Sneak It In

Sometimes what our kids don't know won't hurt them. In fact, it could make them healthier. Have you found it challenging to feed your kids vegetables? Do they fake-vomit at the sight of broccoli and brussels sprouts? Amy and I have figured out how to be strategic in keeping our kids healthy by sneaking in fruits, veggies, and other good things into their meals. They can't tell the difference. The food is delicious and healthy. Here are some ideas:

- Add wheat germ or flaxseed to cereals and oatmeal.

- Add pureed vegetables such as sweet potatoes, squash, broccoli, and cauliflower to muffin and cake mixes.

- Add fruits such as apples, blueberries, and peaches and protein yogurt to waffle and pancake mixes.

- Add vegetables such as peppers, onions, spinach, and mushrooms to eggs.

- Mix green veggies in all of your favorite lasagna, spaghetti, and other casserole dishes.

- Make quinoa pasta instead of oatmeal for breakfast to add extra protein and iron.

Areas of Special Concern for Our Family

Sugar

Most Americans consume too much sugar, perhaps even to the point of being addicted to it. The U.S. Department of Agriculture (USDA) reports that the average American consumes anywhere between *150 to 170 pounds* of simple sugars, also known as refined sugars (this includes glucose, fructose, and sucrose) or simple carbohydrates, in one year! Compare this number to the 4 pounds of sugar the average American consumed less than a hundred years ago. That's a lot of sugar in our system!

Perhaps 150–170 pounds of sugar seems like an astronomical number to you, but think about this. A typical 12-ounce can of soda contains 40 grams, or 10 teaspoons, of sugar. If you drink two Cokes a day, by the end of the week you will have consumed 140 teaspoons of sugar. Let's not forget all the sugar found in doughnuts, cookies, cake, and ice cream, and the hidden sugar (sugar by different names such as high-fructose corn syrup, sucrose, dextrose, glucose, fructose, maltose, and sorbitol) found in salad dressings, hot dogs, canned soups, and bread.

I'm sure you know what happens when your kids eat too many sugary snacks and beverages. They act a little crazy, don't they? Kathleen

DesMaisons is the president and CEO of Radiant Recovery, a nutrition-based addiction recovery program and the author of the book *Little Sugar Addicts*. She has studied the relationship between sugar, health, and behavior and confirms that too much sugar changes our children (and not in a good way). Not only can excess sugar transform your cute, happy child into a teary-eyed monster, but it can also:

- increase the likelihood of cavities
- cause weight gain, because sugar-laden foods are typically high in calories
- increase the chance of your child getting diabetes
- suppress your child's immune system
- promote sugar highs (and related lows)
- promote cravings, because too much sugar raises your blood glucose level, which triggers a spike in insulin

Soda is one of the biggest culprits in the battle against poor health because it contains so much sugar. Public health officials call these drinks liquid candy. Most boys get 15 teaspoons of refined sugar daily, and most girls about 10 teaspoons, from sweetened beverages. According to the Center for Science in the Public Interest, this is the maximum amount of sugar kids should be getting from foods in a day.

According to the National Soft Drink Association (NSDA), consumption of soft drinks is now over 600 12-ounce servings per person per year. Since 1978, soda consumption in the U.S. has tripled for boys and doubled for girls. Soft-drink producers understand the desire kids have for soda, so they amp up their marketing campaigns, often spending billions of dollars to advertise and promote soft drinks.

It's time we rallied against these companies and stopped buying sweetened beverages. Remember, you are in charge of what food and drink comes into your home. Instead of soda, drink water. Make it a priority. Keep fresh water easily accessible to your kids. Buy a water cooler or keep a pitcher of water in your fridge. Carry a water bottle around, and make your kids do the same.

While you may not need to eliminate sugar completely from your family's diet, the key is to eat very few processed foods, sugary snacks, and beverages laden with sugar. Here are some ways to curb the sugar habit in your child's diet:

- Dilute fruit juice with water or drink only 100 percent fruit juice.

- Replace sugary snacks such as cookies and crackers with fruit.

- Eat more natural foods instead of processed and packaged meals and snacks.

- Cook more homemade meals so you can control how much sugar is in each meal.

- Throw out all sugary snacks and treats and replace them with healthier alternatives such as yogurt and protein bars.

Salt

Too much salt is just as bad as too much sugar. The average American consumes 3½ pounds of sodium in a year. That's about 10 times more than the human body requires, which is about 500 milligrams of sodium per day. The Centers for Disease Control recommends that most adults should not consume more than 2,300 mg of sodium. If you are over 40, have high blood pressure, you should lower that to 1,500 mg. The amount is even less for children. The Mayo Clinic submits that kids 4 to 8 years old should consume no more than 1,200 mg of sodium per day. Children 9 years and older can stick with 1,500 mg per day.

Why is excess salt so bad? It can lead to high blood pressure, kidney failure, and strokes. It increases the number of fat cells in your body and makes the ones you already have larger. It makes you more hungry and thirsty, and it slows down your metabolism. Those are just a few reasons to shake the salt from your diet!

In the Parham household, we have seen how easy it is to consume too much salt. This is one reason why we read labels and buy low-salt versions of popular foods. When we reduced our salt intake, our taste buds opened up and we started enjoying food more. It's amazing how pouring on the salt can detract from the natural flavorings in foods. To cut down on our sodium intake, we also stopped going to fast-food restaurants, stopped eating processed foods, and started using spices and chilies to flavor our food.

Fat

Most junk foods and drive-thru restaurant items contain a lot of fat. Not all fat is bad. We need some fat in our diet, but it should be no more than 30 percent of our daily calorie intake. The three basic fats and oils are unsaturated fat, saturated fat, and trans fat/hydrogenated oils. Good fats are unsaturated. We need them for energy and for our bodies to absorb vitamins and other important nutrients. Good fats and oils also help children grow and develop properly. Unsaturated fats are found in such foods as olive oil, canola oil, safflower oil, soybean oil, flax seed, walnuts, peanuts, and almonds.

Saturated fats and trans fats are the bad kind that we need to look out for (read your food labels!). Saturated fats include butter, margarine, shortening, and the fat in animal products such as cheese and meat. While you don't need to eliminate saturated fats completely, you should consume only a limited amount. Saturated fats can contribute to heart disease, clog your veins, and cause central nervous system problems.

Trans fat is created when hydrogen is added to vegetable oil. They help increase the shelf life and flavor of foods. Trans fat is found in many processed foods such as cookies, cakes, crackers, and most fast foods. If you avoid these fats altogether, you will be on your way to better health.

Many fast-food chains and food companies have gone out of their way to lower or eliminate trans fat in their foods. But now another dangerous fat is quickly garnering a lot of attention. Interesterified fat is the new fat to beware of. It is an oil that food scientists have created by moving fatty acids from one triglyceride molecule to another. Recent studies suggest that this type of fat may increase heart-disease risk by lowering HDL (good) cholesterol and raising LDL (bad) cholesterol. They also might increase the risk of type 2 diabetes. So food manufacturers have basically replaced a bad fat with a bad fat.

If you're confused about this, don't worry. The key is not to eat high-fat foods, such as those found in fast-food chains and processed foods and foods that are fried or smothered in butter or oil. Fast food is the kicker. Stop eating it! Did you know that 33 percent of the USDA's top 100 high-fat foods are fast foods? Drive away from the drive-thru. This is by far the quickest way to eliminate bad fats from your diet.

Changing your eating habits around to better your health may seem like an insurmountable task, but it is doable. And you must do it if you want to be healthy and you want your children to be healthy and to reduce their chance of getting certain diseases and illnesses when they get older. I believe there is power in knowledge. Go to your local library and check out some books on how to eat healthier. Here are some we recommend:

- *Eating for Life* by Bill Phillips
- *Betty Crocker's Best of Healthy and Hearty Cooking: More Than 400 Recipes Your Family Will Love*
- *More Healthy Homestyle Cooking: Family Favorites You'll Make Again and Again* by Evelyn Tribole

I like what the Bible says about how we should take care of our bodies, inside and out: "Do you not know that your body is the temple (the very sanctuary) of the Holy Spirit Who lives within you, Whom you have received [as a Gift] from God? You are not your own, you were bought with a price [purchased with a preciousness and paid for, made His own]. So then, honor God and bring glory to Him in your body" (1 Corinthians 6:19-20 AMP).

Take care of your health and take care of your children's health. Show God how much you respect His creation and use your healthy body as a temple to glorify Him.

Plan of Action

- Eat natural. Choose your meals and snacks from fruits, vegetables, lean meats, and whole grains.
- Drink water. It's God's choice of beverage.
- Eat more fiber. Fruit and vegetables are the key.
- Try to balance your meals and snacks with the right amount of carbohydrates, protein, and good fat.
- Eat for one. Don't overestimate your portions. Measure if you have to.

- There is always a healthy alternative for an unhealthy food. Remember the trade game.

- Make sure your family's meals are made with low sugar, low salt, and low (or no) bad fat.

A healthy lifestyle doesn't end simply by eating the right foods. It's about activating your body. It's about getting off the couch and going for a walk, a hike, or a bike ride. It's about doing fun things that will get your blood pumping and your heart rate up. When you couple a good diet with activity, you have a healthy winning combination!

5

Activate Your Kids

When Amy and I speak, I often tell the story about the night a man came by my family's house when I was a teenager. Dressed in a suit and carrying a briefcase, he sat on our living room couch and sold our family on a new phenomenon called cable television. My father immediately bought into his pitch, and the rest of us couldn't have been more thrilled.

When this well-dressed man left, I thought, *Oh boy, we have cable now. We're rich!* I soon discovered I could watch all sorts of things on TV with our new 13-channel selection. I was blown away that I could watch the Atlanta Braves play on TV. I thought cable was the best thing that could have happened to us. But in hindsight, I can see how this new "invention" began to limit our once active lifestyle.

As a little boy—and I'm sure many of you can relate—most of my time outside of school was spent playing outdoors. I don't have many memories of doing things indoors. I rode my bike and played football and basketball with the neighborhood kids. Our birthday parties were outdoors. I sustained many injuries from playing on the swing set or jungle gym. I spent weekends at my grandparents' farm exploring their huge property.

Boy, how things have changed. It's strange being a witness to the digital age. Not that all technology is bad, but it has negatively affected our once active lifestyle. And no, it's not technology's fault. We as parents hold much of the blame for allowing our children to spend more time playing video games than playing in the yard.

The lifestyle of my three boys is much different than mine was. Like any other kid, they want the newest and coolest video games and systems (which seem to pop up every month). They have laptops, iPods, and TVs in their rooms. Since Amy and I have transformed our lifestyle for better health, we've made major changes in this area. We have set firm boundaries and rules in place to ensure that technology does not monopolize our family's time, energy, or health.

Unfortunately, too many parents are not aware (or choose to ignore) how video games, TV, or the Internet have taken dominion over their household. But these things rule our homes. And we are reaping the consequences of that takeover. One major repercussion is obvious: we are continually becoming more sedentary.

A Couch Potato Society

Nielsen's 2009 fourth-quarter "Three Screen Report"—a regular analysis from Nielsen that studies video viewing and related consumer behavior in the U.S.—reveals some sobering statistics. The biggest change in recent years has been that the average American has added more video platforms to their entertainment repertoire. Here's what I mean.

- Each week the typical American watches almost 35 hours of TV; 2 hours of "timeshifted" (DVR) TV; 4 hours of Internet; 22 minutes of online video; and 4 minutes of mobile video.

- 59 percent of Americans now use TV and the Internet simultaneously at least once per month, spending 3.5 hours.

- Americans continue to increase their video use to new levels: TV +1 percent, timeshifting +25 percent, and online video +16 percent.

- Below is the breakdown on how children under the age of 18 spend their time per week on media-related devices:

	Ages 2–11	Ages 12–17
On traditional TV	25:17	23:24
Watching timeshifted TV	1:33	1:15
Using the Internet	0:24	1:21
Watching video on Internet	0:04	0:15
Watching video on a mobile phone	n/a	0:21

Source: The Nielsen Company

The average child spends way too much time sitting. Not only are our children inactive, but they are more likely to indulge in bad eating habits while watching TV or playing video games, causing unnecessary weight gain and health problems.

We need to teach our children to get up and move! It's as simple as that. Exercise is not a means of physical torture or something reserved for gym class. Exercise is being active and moving around. That's all. It's real simple. It can be playing sports, taking dance classes, playing tag in the park, riding bikes, or running around with friends during recess.

The U.S. surgeon general and other leading medical experts recommend that children get an hour of exercise a day. Sadly, this is not happening. Less than one-third of kids aged 6 to 17 get at least 20 minutes of vigorous exercise a day. Why? They're spending all their time watching YouTube videos, listening to their iPods, playing their Wii or DS, or watching TV.

But wait, there's more! According to research by the Discovery Health Channel:

- 50 percent of children do not get enough exercise to develop healthy heart and lungs
- 98 percent of children have at least one heart disease risk
- 20 to 30 percent are already obese

Adults don't fare much better.

- 64 percent don't get enough exercise to maintain healthy heart and lungs
- 24 percent never exercise
- More than 35 percent are overweight

This should be a big "Ouch!" for many of us. Just remember all we talked about in chapter 3. Lead by example. If you don't engage in an active lifestyle, what makes you think your kid will?

The Life-Changing Benefits of Exercise

The obvious plan of attack should be to exercise more as a family. Before we get into creative ways to incorporate a fit and active lifestyle into your home, let me tell you why exercise is necessary. Here are a few of the life-changing benefits of being physically active.

Relieves stress. Regular aerobic exercise releases hormones that give you a sense of well-being and relieve stress.

Alleviates depression. Regular physical activity increases serotonin, a brain chemical that fights negative thoughts and depression.

Boosts mood. Exercise also releases endorphins, powerful chemicals in our brain that give us energy and make us feel good.

Sharpens brainpower. Endorphins also help us focus and sharpen our mind.

Improves self-esteem. When you incorporate regular activity into your life, you take care of yourself and feel better which, in turn, can elevate a stronger sense of self.

Boosts energy. When you are active, your heart rate increases, which gives you extra energy for the rest of your day. Think of exercise as an energy booster.

Benefits overall health. Let's not forget what exercise can do for your health! Do you want your children to have stronger muscles and bones? A leaner body? Less risk of becoming overweight? A decrease in the risk of diseases and medical conditions such as diabetes, high blood pressure, and high cholesterol? Of course you do!

All these benefits should motivate you to get up off the couch, grab your child by the hand, and head outdoors for a nature walk.

What Kind of Exercise Do We Need?

Don't think of exercise as running on a treadmill like a hamster on a wheel. As I mentioned before, exercise can be equated with physical activity. Get off your behind and on your feet moving. It doesn't have to take place in a gym with fancy and scary-looking equipment. It can be any physical activity that gets you breathing harder and raises your heart rate.

There are so many options—from playing a sport to housecleaning to riding a bike to jumping on a trampoline. I like to keep it simple when thinking of family exercise. If you exert energy doing something, you are being active, and that's a good thing.

Remember the saying, "No pain, no gain"? Unfortunately, many people associate exercise with something that will make them hurt, and they shy away from it. After all, who wants to feel pain? But exercise doesn't have to be painful, arduous, or feel like a chore. Exercise can be fun! Riding a bike is fun. Going hiking is fun. Playing catch with your son or daughter is fun. Running around on a beach and swimming is fun.

Rethink exercise as being active and having fun—a perfect combination.

Simple Steps to an Active Lifestyle

Family Power

So what now? If you are a parent who has not embraced physical activity in your home, you can make a change today. I believe incorporating good habits should flow from the head down. Lead your family into the joys, benefits, and fun of exercising. You'll quickly see that the best way for your children to have a fit lifestyle is to make it a family thing.

Amy and I were asked recently to be the masters of ceremonies at a youth triathlon in our area. We were honored to be a part of this inspiring event and enjoyed the experience. I met many wonderful people and came home with fond, lasting memories. What struck me the most was how happy these kids were, even though they were competing so early on a Saturday morning. Many of them looked up to their parents, most of whom were runners themselves. The pattern was obvious. These kids were following their parents' lead.

I like to say that a family that plays together stays together. I admire parents who come home from work and shoot some hoops with their kid in their driveway or who go inline skating with them in the park on the weekends. Spending active time together increases the quality of your relationship and strengthens the bond with your child.

An active family is also a happy family. When we got back from *The Biggest Loser*, we started doing all sorts of fun activities we had never done before with our kids. For instance, when Amy and I won the prize to come home for a day, we took our kids hiking for the first time. It sparked a passion in our family that has continued since.

In one of our early hikes, our youngest son, Rhett, who was not used to exercising, started sweating profusely and complaining how strenuous it was. His voice still rings in my ears, "Dad! Mom! I'm tired! I hurt! My calories hurt!"

Rhett had been hearing us talk about calories so much, he didn't know how to express the extent of his pain other than to say that everything hurt, even his calories. We all had a great laugh that afternoon, and as tired as Rhett was at the start of the hike, he felt like a million bucks toward the end. And he told us how much fun it was!

If I look back at our fondest family memories, I don't remember the times we cleaned our house, took out the trash, played video games, or watched TV. I remember the moments we were together doing something active and fun, from going hiking at the state park to inline skating down the street to playing in the pool at the local YMCA.

Exercise with your kids. Be active with them and build playful memories they'll never forget.

Get Moving

Here are some ideas to activate your family:

- Go for a walk after dinner. If you have young children, put them in a stroller.

- Walk the dog together (if you have one, of course). If not, you can always borrow a friend's or family member's dog that your child loves being around.

- Engage in seasonal activities. Go hiking, in-line skating, canoeing, swimming, or bicycling in the spring, summer, and fall. Try ice-skating or skiing in the winter.

- Do family chores together. Rake the leaves in the backyard with your child. Clean the car. Mow the lawn. Make it fun by charting with gold stars or another kind of treat how many chores your children did.

- Enroll your child in sports classes or fitness groups. See what your school or community offers that your child may be interested in. You may even join a gym that offers fitness programs for the young ones.

- Organize a "dance party" at your house one night. Rally your children to dress up in fancy clothes, put some dance music on the stereo, and spend an hour dancing and being silly with your kids. Younger children particularly love this.

- Go bowling.

- Learn martial arts.

- Have a weekly sports night. Try a new sport each week, such as tennis, golf, skating, and soccer. You've got a lot of options to try out.

- Run or walk for charity. Do some good and get your blood pumping.

- Promote movement in everyday activities. Take the stairs instead of the elevator. Park farther from shopping center entrances. And even if you are watching TV, dance or do jumping jacks during the commercials. Have a contest to see who can do the most.

Motivate Your Child to Be Active

Kids are very different. My boys have different characteristics, personality traits, wants, and needs from each other. And they are motivated in different ways. When it comes to instilling fit habits in your home, you might have to motivate your child more or less than we have to motivate our boys. Some kids will have no problem with you telling them to drop the video-game controller and go outside to play. Others will groan, protest, and voice their annoyance every step of the way.

Also, children have different fitness levels. If your child is inactive, simply taking a walk with him or having her help around the house will help break this pattern. Slowly ease your children into physical activity. If they are moderately active, challenge them. Have their friends come over to play football or basketball. Explore new types of exercise with them. Find a list of activities at school or in the community and review them with your child. See what interests him or her.

However you decide to get your family up and moving, set a positive example and make sure you are having fun as well. If you're not happy being active, I guarantee that your children will likewise be unhappy.

If your child is overweight or refuses to be active, don't fall into the trap of enablement. You enable your child when you allow him (even if you have good intentions) to do things that are harmful or irresponsible. This happens when you rescue him from a situation instead of letting him deal with the consequences or let him get away with things instead of holding him accountable for his actions.

I know many parents who refuse to encourage their overweight child to be more physically active simply because their child expresses no interest. Some parents can even relate to their kid's problem because they, too, were overweight as children and understand the hurt that comes from the ridicule of classmates. But if their style of managing the situation is to simply soothe the child and say, "Everything's okay," they are walking the thin line of enablement.

Empower your kids instead. Be the household motivator to change unhealthy behaviors or patterns instead of enabling your children to walk a permanent path of poor health. As a parent, you want the best for your children, so you need to be firm and be aware of the consequences of a sedentary lifestyle and poor nutrition habits.

Sure, it's going to be hard for many kids in the beginning. They will whine. They will cry. They will complain. They may even be resentful. It's okay! Change for any human being is uncomfortable.

But this is a great teaching moment. This is how your children learn that creating a future worth having requires doing the work. It requires making some changes. But it also can be fun and engaging.

Remember, if you want your children to

- feel better about themselves
- maintain a healthy weight
- build strong bones, muscles, and joints
- do better in school
- hit the path of adulthood with healthy habits
- sleep better

then adjust your current lifestyle to be more active. Keep it fun. Keep it positive. And keep it for the rest of your life!

Plan of Action
- Set a good example. Your children will follow your lead.
- Limit TV, computer, and video-game time.

- Promote activity, not exercise. Just get your kids off the couch and moving. And remember, all activity counts.

- Involve your entire family in physical activity to build a strong bond.

- Get your kids into the great outdoors as much as possible. Fresh air can do wonders for your child.

- Be the parent. Set rules and limits and do not enable your kids by letting them do what they want. Empower them for a healthy and fit future.

We know that in today's fast-paced culture, families are busier than ever. Incorporating good health into your life means reexamining your priorities and figuring out how you can manage your time more wisely. We are living proof that it's possible to be and stay healthy, even when life is full of demands and responsibilities.

6

Finding Balance

One thing about life never changes—it is always changing! You finally get settled in your new home, and your husband gets a new job in another state. You finally have some peace and quiet home from work one day, and your child gets sick at school and needs you to come get her. You are thrilled about your dream job, and a floundering economy forces you to shut down your business.

Change is also a constant in our health lifestyle. Does this sound familiar? You get excited about eating right and getting more exercise, but a stomach virus infects your house, and your family is stuck at home for days. Or after a solid number of weeks prioritizing your nutrition needs, your company sends you on a business trip, and you have to leave the kids with the hubby who thinks pizza is one of the four food groups, and you find yourself having to get by on airport food for a few days.

If we aren't careful, these things can trip us up in our journey to good health. The key to having balance in the midst of life's changes, bumps, twists, and detours is maintaining the right perspective. We can't be so rigid that we don't allow for flexibility sometimes. Life happens! If we let setbacks stop us from moving forward, then we'll never accomplish our goals.

Most of you parents—especially you mothers—have the best intentions when it comes to planning and organizing. We would love nothing more than for our days, weeks, months, and years to go as smoothly as we have planned them. But that's not going to happen. We need to expect the unexpected. When life puts a wrench in our plans, we need to regroup, reevaluate priorities and goals, and forge on ahead. Finding the balance between structure and flexibility is the goal we should strive toward.

Keys to Building Structure in Your Healthy Home

One thing that has helped Phillip and me win (most of the time) the battle of providing a health structure in our household is learning how to plan. Before our health transformation, we were "fly by the seat of our pants" kind of people. Our personalities are such that we tended to do everything at the last minute. If someone asked me on Wednesday what my plans for the weekend were, I wouldn't have thought that far ahead. More oft than not, I would have my weekend plans figured out sometime on Friday.

Living this way caused us to waste time and money, not to mention the cost of bad eating habits. I used to think about the family's dinner plans on my way home from work, and my solution usually involved ordering takeout or getting dinner at the drive-thru. Definitely not a healthy choice for a healthy family.

Now we think and plan ahead so we know what our family will be eating for the week as well as when we will squeeze in exercise. When you plan ahead, it helps you overcome some of the bad last-minute choices you might be tempted to make.

I also notice that when I plan ahead, I manage my time more efficiently. We are all on a time budget. We all have 24 hours in our day. What we do with that 24 hours makes the difference between success and failure.

Here are some planning tips we use to save our family time and money and balance a healthy lifestyle with life's demands.

Plan Your Meals

We plan our meals for two weeks because Phillip and I get paid biweekly. We found planning according to our financial budget makes the most sense for us. Planning this much time in advance may seem like a lot of work, and initially it will be, but it really does save so much time down the road. You'll never have to think about what you'll be eating on any given day or plan unnecessary trips to the grocery store.

Phillip and I write down breakfast, lunch, snacks, and dinner for 14 days and estimate the amount of food we need to buy for those two weeks. For example, if we know we're going to have eggs every morning, we buy enough for 14 days. If our kids will be eating cereal for two weeks, we buy enough to last for that time. Of course certain items, such as milk, you have to shop for every week or cannot buy in bulk.

We divide our shopping list into what we can buy at the wholesale store and what we can buy at the grocery store. We use the wholesale store for such things as eggs, oatmeal, cereal, frozen boneless chicken breasts, frozen tilapia and salmon, quinoa pasta, brown rice, and whole-wheat pasta (see appendix A for our complete shopping list). The items for the grocery store might be specialty spices or herbs (such as cilantro), and rotisserie chicken, bread, and fresh fruit and vegetables.

Cook Ahead

After we do our shopping, we decide what meals or snacks we can make ahead of time so that we have them available when we need them. Chicken, beef, turkey, brown rice, quinoa, sweet potatoes, and steamed vegetables are good to prepare up to a week ahead of when you'll use them.

In the Parham household, we reserve Sundays to cook our meals. We find this day works best for us, but choose whatever day works for you. After we get home from church, we spend a couple of hours in the kitchen preparing our meals for the week. The time we spend together is also a great opportunity to share quality time as a family. We are all together, doing something good for our health, and having fun in the process. The most time-consuming part of this cooking-ahead project is the actual cooking. But once that's done, you'll see how easy meal and snack time really can be.

We also cut up raw fruit and vegetables and put them in individual plastic bags so that they are readily available for snacks and school lunches for our kids. Then we divvy up foods such as rice, pasta, quinoa, steamed veggies, and meats in individual plastic containers so that we have them ready to take with us during the week for lunch or save in the fridge for dinnertime.

We always have plenty of chicken prepared because it's one of the easiest ingredients to whip up a quick and healthy meal. You can make a chicken wrap or a chicken salad, for instance. You can also throw some veggies in with chicken and serve over whole-wheat pasta or you can make a chicken and rice casserole.

We also like to make what we call a "healthy snack" basket for our boys. If your kids are anything like ours, as soon as they come home from school, they head straight to the kitchen to grab whatever they can find to snack on. We like to make sure they have the healthiest options available to them. We take such items as protein bars, Kashi granola bars, blue corn tortilla chips, almonds, pistachios, popcorn, oranges, apples, bananas, and pears and put them in a basket in the pantry so our boys can choose a snack that is "legal." We divide the basket into individual portions so our boys know how much they can eat. We also make sure we have plenty of snacks in the fridge, such as string cheese, grapes, and veggies.

Another way that helps me plan and balance my time demands is making my kids' lunches at a certain time. I found it works best for me to prepare their lunches while they're having their afternoon snack. Taking care of this task the day before eliminates the morning rush.

To save time, we have also come to rely on our slow cooker. We got three of them for our wedding over 20 years ago and didn't start using them until recently. They are a lifesaver! The slow cooker is great for making soups, sauces, and stews. You can throw your ingredients in the pot in the morning, and when you get home from work, voilà!—dinner is served. It's such a relief to come home after a long, hard day and not have to think about what you're going to have for dinner.

Getting Active

So how do we maintain balance in our homes when it comes to fitness? With the busy lives we lead, we have to squeeze in activity with our boys any time we can. They love playing sports, so we make sure to keep them involved through the year in a sports activity in the community or at school.

We make activity a part of our everyday lives. If we're going to the mall or the grocery store as a family, we park in a spot far from the entrance. If one of our boys has baseball or soccer practice, we take the other children and walk around the field with them.

We also plan weekend activities that are fun and physical. Our hometown of Greenville, North Carolina, has a beautiful downtown area that offers a multitude of family-oriented street festivals, races, outdoor markets, and other goings-on. We love taking our kids there and walking from one end of Main Street to the other. An old-fashioned toy store and a general store are at one end. At the other end, you'll find a huge suspension bridge over a river. Our kids enjoy wading in the water and climbing on the big rocks that line the riverbed. We have spent many weekends walking that area and exploring the river. Our boys love it, and Phillip and I do too! This is just one of the many ways we incorporate activity into our family life.

Just Say No

Sometimes (more times than not, I've found) balancing good health in family life means eliminating or saying no to activities or hobbies that promote unhealthy habits. Remember our beef with TV and video games in chapter 5? I'm sure you'll agree that most kids today spend too much time on media-driven technology. Video games, television, and computer games take up a lot of valuable time and prevent us from being as fit as we could be.

As I mentioned earlier, our family is constantly aware of our time budget. Through some of the tips we've shown you, we have saved a ton of time (and money) planning our meals. We also saved a ton of time— time that we use toward physical activity—when we limited how many hours a week our kids spent watching TV or playing video games.

I'm not naïve. I know that my kids could probably spend the whole day in front of the big screen if I let them. And if I didn't have responsibilities, I just might be tempted to sit on the couch and watch movies all day. But this is not what builds a healthy lifestyle for my kids or for me.

We need to monitor what our kids are doing and set boundaries at home for how they spend their time. It may seem like we're the bad guys policing their every move, but guess what? We're the parents. We get to make the decisions. We get to tell them what is best for them. And finding time to be active is better for them than turning into TV zombies.

I remember when my kids were toddlers and it came time to feed them, I would put them in their high chairs, plop some food on their tray, and turn on *Veggie Tales*. I was so exhausted (probably because of my poor diet and lack of exercise) that I wanted the television to babysit them for a little while. I didn't think it was that bad. Certainly there were worse things I could have done. I look back at that time and realize that I was establishing patterns that would be difficult for them to break in the future.

If you are the mother of a toddler (or two), don't fall prey to this temptation. By training your kids to be entertained by television while eating, they will continue to engage in that pattern as they get older. And while you can break the pattern when they grow up, it's much harder than if you had never set the pattern to begin with.

So many things in this world consume our time and do not benefit us. Think about your own lifestyle. How much time do you spend mindlessly surfing the Web? How much time do you spend talking on the phone with your girlfriends? How much time do you spend watching football? How much time do you spend on Facebook? Get the picture? We must hold ourselves accountable for how wisely we use our time in the same way we enforce that behavior with our children.

When you see your kids lounging around the TV on a Saturday afternoon, shut it off and tell them to play outside. Instead of seeing a movie as a family, go bowling or miniature golfing. Instead of socializing on the Internet while your kids play video games, get out of the house and go for a nature walk together in a nearby park.

Sadly, we have become a society that spends a great amount of time doing things that don't require us to exert ourselves physically. While we can't change that culturally, we can change it in our families. Give your kids a budgeted amount of time for certain activities, such as watching TV and playing video games. Set the same standards for yourself.

It is possible to maintain good health in your family even when your schedule looks crazy and your to-do list is a mile long. It just requires making sacrifices and substituting unhealthy activities with healthy ones. You have the choice to steward your time wisely or poorly. The choice is yours. Honor God, respect yourself, and build a healthy family by making good decisions that will give you lasting rewards.

Get Your ZZZZZZZs

Make a good night's sleep a priority. Sleep is critical in so many ways. The Harvard Women's Health Watch reported in 2008 that sleep should not be shortchanged. Here are a few reasons why getting 7–8 hours of sleep (for adults) is so important.

- Sleep improves your memory and helps you learn better.
- Chronic sleep deprivation may cause weight gain.

- Sleep debt contributes to a greater tendency to fall asleep during the daytime, which may cause preventable accidents, mishaps, and errors.

- Sleep loss may result in irritability, impatience, inability to concentrate, and moodiness.

- Serious sleep disorders have been linked to hypertension, increased stress-hormone levels, and irregular heartbeat.

- Sleep deprivation affects your immune system, including the activity of the body's killer cells.

We don't need a plethora of studies to back this up. You know what happens when you don't get enough sleep. You're groggy. You're cranky. You're moody. And you just don't feel good. When we don't get enough rest, there is no doubt that our performance at work, school, or even as a parent is affected negatively. If you don't get enough sleep, you are apt to be less motivated to influence positive health changes in your family.

Kids need sleep too! The average kid has a busy day. She goes to school, runs around with friends, goes to extracurricular events after school, and does homework. By the end of her day, she needs a chance to unwind and prepare for the next day of much the same.

Our kids can function best only if they get enough sleep. Most experts say that kids between the ages of 5 and 12 need about 10 or 11 hours of sleep per night. Does your child get that much? If not, it may be time to send them to bed earlier.

Don't Be So Hard on Yourself

Don't feel overwhelmed at the task of finding balance. We all have days when nothing goes right. Our best laid plans get foiled sometimes. Don't worry. It's normal. Maybe you can't cook ahead because you have to work overtime, or you can't exercise for a week because you have the flu.

Stuff will happen sometimes that is outside of our control. Go with the flow as best as you can, and when things get back on track, get back on your structured routine. Don't give up simply because you get sidetracked for a bit. Pick up right where you left off.

It doesn't matter how excellent you are at following a routine once or twice; it matters most if you do it consistently. I've found that many people are extreme when it comes to changing their life habits. They go from 0 to 60 overnight. Though they never worked out a day in their life, they plan on working out two hours a day. Though they've had poor nutrition habits for many years, they vow to give up sugar, salt, and fat for the rest of their life.

The same applies to families. Don't throw your kids into a different (and revolutionary) routine and expect things to work smoothly at first. Ease them into eating better and being more active. Take this new adventure one step at a time. If you choose to use an extreme approach right off the bat, I guarantee you will run out of steam and quit the whole thing.

If you have to go to the drive-thru, choose the healthiest item on the menu (such as a chicken salad with low-fat dressing). If you get sick or hurt and can't take your kids exercising for a few days, take the time to recover, and as soon as you feel better, take them for a jog around the neighborhood. A balanced, healthy lifestyle is not a perfect one. It's merely consistent most of the time. That's all you can ask for.

At this point, you might be feeling bad for some of the unhealthy habits you've let creep into your home. Some of you may even be condemning yourself for your actions. You may think that you've let poor health infiltrate your family for so long, it seems impossible to get them on the right track. The first thing you must do is forgive yourself. I like what author Maya Angelou said:

> I don't know if I continue, even today, always liking myself. But what I learned to do many years ago was to forgive myself. It is very important for every human being to forgive herself or himself because if you live, you will make mistakes—it is inevitable. But once you do and you see the mistake, then you forgive yourself and say, "Well, if I'd known better I'd have done better," that's all. So you say to people who you think you may have injured, "I'm sorry," and then you say to yourself, "I'm sorry." If we all hold on to the mistake, we can't see our own glory in the mirror because we have the mistake between our faces and the mirror; we can't see what we're capable of being. You can ask forgiveness of others, but in the end the real forgiveness is in one's own self.

I know that sometimes forgiving yourself can seem like an insurmountable mountain to climb. I want to encourage you that it is possible! Many times I have found it difficult to show myself some mercy and grace over the poor choices I made for myself and my family. At times, just thinking about making changes made me feel tired and confused. I was so overwhelmed, I didn't know where to start.

After we came home from the ranch and realized the obstacles we had to face to transform our family's lifestyle, we were initially discouraged. But we fought the battle one day at a time, one step at a time. And dear reader, I am filled with hope and confidence that you, too, can do the same for your family.

Plan of Action

- Plan your meals ahead of time so you can avoid last-minute, unhealthy food choices.

- Fit active time into your daily routine wherever you can. Be creative. Any movement works!

- Eliminate or limit any household activity (such as watching TV or playing video games) that wastes time and doesn't provide long-term, healthy benefits.

- Get 7–8 hours of sleep (10–11 for kids) to function at your best.

In the next chapter, we're going to talk about the major steps you need to take to change your family into a healthy and fit one. Through reading this next chapter, you'll be put at ease knowing that change is not only possible, but something that will happen if you follow the process we've taken ourselves.

As two full-time working parents raising a family of three boys, one of whom has a disability, we know it can be tough to maintain healthy habits in the home. But we are living proof that it can be done, and we know very well the awesome benefits that can be reaped from making better choices.

Getting Started

---------------- A Word from Amy ----------------

Dump the Junk

It's time to take the next steps to permanent, healthy change in your new lifestyle!

When it comes to being healthy, I believe your primary concern needs to be your diet. You are what you eat, after all. Your first course of action is to clean out your refrigerator and pantry of unhealthy foods, snacks, and drinks. This may be a hard task for you, but it will be especially traumatic for your children if they have been addicted to sugar, salt, and fatty foods. You must be prepared for the backlash. Stand strong, parents, I know you can do this!

Have you ever seen an old war movie where a soldier gets shot in the leg and gangrene sets in? What do the medics do to his leg? They cut it off. If they didn't, the poison would affect the whole body and he would likely die. Amputation is the only way to keep the rest of the body healthy. Cleaning out your pantry and kitchen has a similar effect. You are cutting out the "gangrene" in your home so that your family can be healthy.

When we did this after we got back from the ranch, our kids were not happy campers. This was one task we didn't do gradually. We threw all the bad stuff away and replaced it with healthy food the same day. The boys didn't stand a chance. There was no time to beg Mom and Dad to keep the Little Debbie cakes. Before they knew what happened, Little Debbie was long gone. This was part of our healthy-healing process. The quicker your family realizes that you are serious about making a change, the faster they will adjust to the idea.

You might think this is extreme. Isn't moderation the key? Shouldn't we be able to have just a bite of chocolate cake? Or a serving of nacho chips? Or a little bowl every now and then of sugary cereal? While we believe self-control is essential and deprivation is not the way to go for the long-term, we also know how critical the start of your transformation is. At this point you need to take some drastic steps to get on the fast track to a healthier you. This is especially true if you have spent most of your life eating junk food and processed meals.

If you don't have unhealthy foods in the house, you will be less tempted to eat them. And temptation is a big deal when you start making major changes in your eating habits. So, is this an extreme action? Perhaps. But it worked for our family, and I'm confident it will work for yours.

Let's get started. Go through your refrigerator, drawers, pantry, closets—anyplace where food is stored—and throw out the following items. If you feel guilty about throwing food away, you can donate it to a local food pantry or shelter.

- Anything that is processed, including processed lunch meats, margarine, processed cheese, white rice, white pasta, white breads, instant foods (canned soups, macaroni and cheese, boxed meals), sweets (cookies, cakes, ice cream), and snacks (crackers and chips)
- Anything that has a long shelf life
- Anything that has refined or high-fructose sugar or has ingredients that you cannot pronounce
- Anything that is *not* natural or minimally processed
- All sugary drinks and sodas

When you're done, you may find that you don't have any food left in the house. This is a good sign that you're on the right track! The less bad stuff you have, the more room you have to replace it with good stuff.

Now it's time to go shopping. You have a clean slate in your kitchen, and this is your opportunity to make a fresh start. Below is a list of what Phil and I consider our staple foods, and we always keep plenty around to whip up meals and snacks. You can also pull from the comprehensive shopping list in appendix A. This list includes items we used on *The Biggest Loser* as well as a few favorites of our own.

Copy this list and take it with you to the grocery store. Obviously, you don't have to purchase everything on the list nor is this list meant to be comprehensive. You can add healthy items that you and your family enjoy eating. For example, kiwi fruit is not on the list, but if you and your family like it, buy it. These lists are merely a guide for healthy choices you can use to stock your kitchen and pantry.

- Old-fashioned oatmeal. Use this instead of the instant varieties. Oatmeal is easy to make and one of the best foods you can eat in the morning. It's packed with fiber, and you can mix it with honey, cinnamon, fruit, flaxseed, or nuts.

- Canned beans (pinto, red, chickpeas, kidney, black, take your pick). Beans are low in fat and high in fiber, calcium, and iron.

- Fresh and frozen vegetables. They are easy to make steamed or cooked in a little bit of extra virgin olive oil. We especially love spinach.

- Fresh fruit. We always have fresh fruit available because it's the perfect snack. It's prepackaged by God in a perfect size.

- Brown rice. We love the kind that you boil in a bag. We mix our rice with salsa and hummus and vegetables. It is filling and delicious.

- Mustard and salsa. These are two great condiments we always use. I love fresh salsa and make it myself when I can. I switched from mayo to mustard and have never looked back.

- Tuna. If I'm in a hurry, I can put a package of tuna in my lunch sack and head out the door. I mix it with mustard, olive oil, and chickpeas when I put it in a salad. It has tons of protein.

- Eggs. We always have eggs around. They are great scrambled or boiled and chopped up into salads.

- Hummus. We make our own hummus, but it's just as easy to buy premade hummus, especially when you're just getting started. It's great to use as a spread or in a dip.

- Lean protein such as chicken, turkey, and fish. Buy frozen or put fresh in your freezer if you don't plan to use it right away.

- Olive oil. This is the best kind for cooking and sautéing.

Planning Your Meals

As I mentioned in chapter 6, we make our meals two weeks in advance. I highly recommend you do the same, especially when you begin the "Challenge." This is another strategy to help jump-start your health transformation.

In the following pages, I'll provide you with two weeks' worth of breakfast, lunch, dinner, and snack ideas that you can use in planning your menu. If you prefer, you can create your own plan...as long as it's healthy.

Include your kids in making the menus. I know my kids love spaghetti, tacos, and meat loaf, so I try to include those items (healthy versions, of course) on the menu almost every week. It beats hearing "Oh, no. Chicken again?" at dinnertime.

If you need some help planning your menu, here are some great cookbooks and additional resources we have used that might be helpful to you:

- *Cooking Light: The Essential Dinner Tonight Cookbook* by Editors of *Cooking Light* magazine

- *The Weeknight Survival Cookbook: How to Make Healthy Meals in 10 Minutes* by Dena Irwin

- *The Biggest Loser Family Cookbook: Budget-Friendly Meals Your Whole Family Will Love* by Devin Alexander and *The Biggest Loser* Experts and Cast with Melissa Roberson

- *Hungry Girl: Recipes and Survival Strategies for Guilt-Free Eating in the Real World* by Lisa Lillien

The following books are great tools for determining the calorie content of various foods: *The Biggest Loser Complete Calorie Counter: The Quick and Easy Guide to Thousands of Foods from Grocery Stores and Popular Restaurants* by Cheryl Forberg and *The Biggest Loser* Experts and Cast, and *The Calorie King Calorie, Fat, and Carbohydrate Counter* by Allan Borushek.

Keep in mind that we are not dieticians. The meals and snacks below are based on what our nutritionists suggested that we eat and what we know works for us. Whatever you decide to eat throughout the day, remember the three keys to determining healthy food choices:

- Make sure 90 percent of your food choices are whole, fresh, and natural (fruits, vegetables, lean meats, and whole grains).
- Stick with the correct portion sizes.
- Eat the right balance of protein, carbohydrates, and fats.

Week 1

Breakfast Ideas

- Ezekiel-bread French toast (Ezekiel bread dipped in egg whites and cooked on a skillet) topped with fresh berries and sugar-free syrup (we like the *Smuckers* brand)
- Old-fashioned (whole oat) oatmeal (you can add diced apples, nuts, cinnamon, xylitol, sugar-free syrup, raisins) and scrambled egg whites
- Veggie omelet (with egg whites, mushrooms, spinach, onions, tomatoes, bell peppers) and whole-wheat toast
- Scrambled egg whites with turkey sausage, mozzarella cheese, red peppers, and onions and a Kashi GOLEAN waffle with sugar-free syrup
- Turkey bacon or sausage and cereal (All-Bran, Kashi GO-LEAN Crunch, Cheerios, and Shredded Wheat are some of our favorites) with skim milk, almond milk, or soy milk
- Egg-white sandwich with turkey bacon on light wheat bread with a tomato or salsa (or both)
- Turkey bacon, egg whites, and wheat toast with sugar-free jelly or fruit

Lunch Ideas

- Tomatoes stuffed with tuna that has been mixed with three-pepper mustard
- Grilled chicken, sweet potato, and asparagus or cauliflower

- Grilled-chicken tortillas with salsa, spinach, and Laughing Cow cheese
- Spinach salad made with spinach, mushrooms, tomatoes, turkey-bacon pieces, and topped with raspberry vinaigrette
- Whole-wheat pasta salad tossed with cherry tomatoes, balsamic vinaigrette dressing, spinach, and kidney beans
- Chicken sandwich with light wheat bread and mustard with carrots and broccoli

Dinner Ideas

- Salmon salad with spring-mix greens, almonds, raisins or dried cranberries, mandarin oranges, tomatoes, mushrooms, and cranberry mustard
- Grilled tilapia with salsa, steamed carrots and broccoli, and brown rice
- Chicken taco salad with chicken, lettuce, blue corn tortilla chips, tomatoes, corn, black beans, and light cheddar cheese with salsa
- Turkey burger with mustard and sweet-potato fries (spray slices of sweet potato with Pam, brush them with honey, and sprinkle a dash of cayenne pepper; bake)
- Chicken salad (chicken-breast chunks, kidney beans, red peppers, and spinach mixed together with a little parmesan cheese)
- Spinach salad with mushrooms and balsamic vinaigrette
- Ground-turkey taco salad (ground turkey, low-sodium taco seasoning, lettuce, salsa, tomatoes, and light cheddar cheese)
- Chicken noodle soup (chicken broth, carrots, celery, and chicken seasoned to taste) and side green salad

Week 2

Breakfast Ideas

- Breakfast burrito made with low-carb wheat wrap, egg

whites, red and green peppers, onions, and mushrooms and sprinkled with low-sodium mozzarella

- Ground-turkey scramble made with ground turkey, egg whites, spinach, red peppers, garlic powder, and salt substitute, served with a slice of light wheat toast
- Breakfast smoothie (water, ice, almond milk, one scoop protein powder, and two tablespoons powdered peanut butter)
- Crunchy oatmeal (old-fashioned oatmeal sweetened with truvia or xylitol, and topped with almonds, walnuts, and dried cranberries)
- Amy McMuffin (whole-wheat English muffin with egg whites, slice of Swiss cheese, and slice of turkey bacon)
- The Quickie (cup of yogurt mixed with protein powder and sprinkled with berries and granola)
- Whole-wheat pancakes with fruit jam and served with turkey bacon

Lunch Ideas

- Peanut butter sandwich made with natural peanut butter and all-fruit jam on light wheat bread
- Grilled chicken, brown rice, and broccoli
- Black beans and brown rice served with steamed veggies
- Chicken salad with spinach, tomatoes, chicken, carrots, and cranberry mixed with three-pepper mustard
- Grilled chicken, brown rice, yellow squash, and zucchini
- Summer salad made with spring mix, grilled chicken breast, strawberries, bleu-cheese crumbles, almonds, and balsamic vinaigrette
- Turkey wrap made with sun-dried tomato, low-carb wrap, spinach, turkey deli meat, mushrooms, tomatoes, and cranberry mustard

Dinner Ideas

- Ground-turkey meat loaf made with ground turkey, old-fashioned oatmeal, onions, green peppers, salt-free seasoning, and sugar-free ketchup with a side of steamed yellow squash, onions, and carrots

- Ground-turkey chili made with ground turkey, chili powder, chopped canned tomatoes, kidney beans, onion, and salt substitute

- Turkey burgers on flatbread wheat buns with onions, mustard, tomato, and lettuce with hummus and carrots

- Mexican turkey burgers (ground-turkey patties seasoned with low-sodium taco seasoning and served over lettuce and tomatoes with salsa and blue corn tortilla chips)

- Turkey meatballs (turkey mixed with onion flakes and salt-free seasoning) with steamed broccoli and mashed potatoes (made with low-sodium chicken broth, salt substitute, minced garlic, and Fage yogurt)

- Whole-wheat spaghetti with homemade spaghetti sauce (chopped canned tomatoes, tomato paste, mushrooms, olive oil, oregano, black pepper, and salt substitute); top with leftover turkey meatballs

- Turkey-meatball soup (canned tomatoes, low-sodium chicken broth, corn, black beans, carrots, jalapenos, black pepper, red pepper flakes, and salt substitute)

Snack Ideas

- Almonds and an apple
- Laughing Cow cheese with Wasa crackers
- Orange with a rice cake
- One-half peanut butter sandwich on light wheat bread
- Banana with one teaspoon of almond butter
- Greek yogurt with berries and xylitol
- Boiled egg with grapefruit

- Air-popped popcorn with almonds (we like to add Tabasco sauce)
- Yogurt with granola
- Carrots and hummus
- Cottage cheese and peaches
- String cheese and grapes
- Celery and peanut butter
- Mixed nuts and berries
- Blue corn tortilla chips with Laughing Cow cheese mixed with salsa and Tabasco sauce

Adding Activity

The final step in getting started on your healthy lifestyle is to schedule time for more activity. Have a family meeting and ask your kids what kinds of things they like to do. If they are unsure, offer suggestions such as hiking, basketball, cycling, swimming, and running. Then let them determine when and what you will plan to do together. Getting your children involved in the decision-making process will make it easier to incorporate activity into your lifestyle because they will be excited about it.

If you have a family calendar, take it out and plan one active family time per week. Then carve out time in your schedule to do smaller-scale activities with your children—such as playing outside together, walking around the block, or going to the park—and do those a few times a week.

Now that you know so much more about what it takes to create and maintain a healthy lifestyle for your family, it's time to start the "Challenge." We believe in you and know that your desire to lead your family toward a healthier and fitter future will benefit you in more ways than you can imagine.

Part 2

Your Daily
Fitness Challenge

For the next 90 days, we are going to walk with your family each day as you progress on this fitness journey. You'll learn, be inspired, and get challenged as you make your way toward better health.

Let's refresh some of what you've learned so far. You understand the importance of maintaining good health habits in your family so you can prevent illnesses, diseases, have more energy, and feel better overall. You know that you need to eat to live, not eat because you're struggling emotionally or simply because it tastes good. You also have to eat the right foods—natural instead of processed.

You realize that including regular activity in your day is essential. As we like to say, sometimes you just gotta get up off the couch and start moving. Plan fun activities as a family so you can spend time and get healthy together. We also gave you some tips to organize your life so that health is a priority. By now you can see that good health is something you can manage even with a busy lifestyle. Most of all, you understand that your kids are watching you, so it's vital that you take care of your health first so they can follow your lead.

Throughout these 90 challenges, we will come alongside to encourage you as you move into a new, healthier you. Each day will be a new adventure where you will learn more and feel better about yourself.

These challenges are divided into nine categories and include the following sections:

> **Something to Think About**—a challenge that will inspire, motivate, and educate you on the path to better health

> **Something to Talk About**—three questions that you can discuss with your family that are specific to the challenge

> **Tip of the Day**—health tips, because taking care of ourselves is a constant learning process

Read these challenges with your children at the breakfast or dinner table. Make it a time to discuss your feelings and thoughts and bond as a family. Remember, this is a challenge for the whole family, and it will be a victory for all of you as well when you make the changes.

Most of all, we are so proud you've decided to start this journey with us. We know you can lead your family into making better health choices and maintaining solid health habits. We are confident that you will soon see positive changes in your family's physical, mental, and emotional health as you start taking better care of your body. You will be amazed at the results!

Let's get started.

Dream Big!

The *Amazing Fitness Adventure for Your Kids* is about dreaming, believing, and achieving. It's time that you and your family grab hold of life as God intended. It's time to get inspired and soar into the future. Know that anything is possible!

DAY 1—A NEW START

A Word from Amy

Something to Think About

You know that feeling you get on the first day of school? It's exciting, but also a little scary. You're starting a new class, getting new teachers, and having new adventures. I remember my first day of kindergarten. I hid behind my mom because I was so shy. As I looked around from behind her skirt, I noticed a cool kitchen area in the corner. And it was just my size.

Although I was still a little afraid, I wanted to play with that kitchen set. The desire became greater than my fear. I got up my courage and ran over to the adorable kitchen. Guess what? The fear went away.

Today might seem like that kind of day for you. It's the beginning of "Your Daily Fitness Challenge," and you are making the choice to be healthier. It may be a little scary for you. That's completely normal. We are all afraid of new things. But like me wanting to play with the kitchen set, I hope the desire to not let anything hold you back from your dreams will motivate you to keep going.

God designed us to have big dreams for our lives. He doesn't want anything (not even extra weight) to hold us back. Just as our parents want to make sure that we have everything we need to succeed, so does God. Come with me and let's *dream*!

Something to Talk About

1. What are some things you want to do with your life? Maybe you want to travel, get a particular job, or have a family. Make a list of those things.

2. Now look at your list and identify things you might not be able to do if you aren't strong, fit, and healthy.

3. Think about something you did that, at first, made you feel very afraid. How did you overcome your fear?

Tip of the Day

Whenever you start to reach for that bottle of soda, remember that

99

the sugar in it will give you energy for a minute, but it will quickly cause you to crash and feel very tired. Drink water instead.

DAY 2—DAYDREAMERS UNITE!

A Word from Amy

Something to Think About

Have you ever been accused of daydreaming in class? Maybe you were thinking about what you were going to do after school. Maybe you were thinking about scoring the winning run at the baseball game. It doesn't matter what you daydream about, what matters is that you are taken away to another place and into a world of possibilities.

Many times we get in trouble when we daydream, but today I'm giving you permission to daydream with me for a minute. I want you to think about your future. What do you want to do when you grow up? I believe that God often gives us a clue about our future in what we daydream about the most. It's our job to play detective and figure out what that plan is.

Get a picture in your mind about what that will look like. What do you see? When you think about your future, I hope you see yourself doing big and mighty things. I hope you won't set any limits on what you can do. When you daydream, know that if you make good choices and don't give up, you can make those daydreams real!

Something to Talk About

1. How important do you think your health is in making your dreams a reality?

2. What steps can you take to make sure you are healthy?

3. What kinds of things do you daydream about? Talk about them as a family. Encourage each other as you share.

Tip of the Day

Rest is an important part of being healthy. When you get plenty of sleep every night, you are able to think more clearly and have more energy. When your parents set a bedtime for you, it's because they want to you to feel good the next day. So don't stay up late playing video games or watching TV. Get a good night's sleep instead.

DAY 3—MAKING THE RIGHT CHOICE

A Word from Amy

Something to Think About

When I was a little girl, my mother owned an ice cream parlor. The cool thing about that was I could have ice cream anytime I wanted. The bad thing about that was also that I could have ice cream anytime I wanted. Because of making bad choices, I ate too much ice cream and before I knew it, my clothes wouldn't fit anymore. I was chubby.

Being overweight caused me to feel bad about myself. Some of the kids started to make fun of me, and it made me feel sad and lonely. I wasn't as outgoing as I had been, and I didn't participate in activities that I once enjoyed because I was too self-conscious.

I'm not telling you this to make you feel sorry for me. I'm telling you this because you have the power to make good or bad choices in your life. Your choices make the difference between whether you see your dreams come true or not.

I encourage you to remember that you have the power, every day, to decide whether you are going to do the right thing. And I believe that you will choose the right things so you can live your dreams!

Something to Talk About

1. How have your bad choices in the past affected your life? For example, maybe you didn't study for a test and got a bad grade. How can you make better choices in the future?

2. What are some good choices you can make where your health is concerned?

3. Think about the dreams you talked about in yesterday's reading. Discuss some good choices you can make that will help those dreams come true.

Tip of the Day

Substituting mustard for mayo is an easy change that can make a difference in your health. Mustard has virtually no calories or fat while mayo is high in fat and calories. Simple choices matter!

DAY 4—GOOD THINGS TAKE TIME

A Word from Amy

Something to Think About

Thirteen-year-old Jordan Romero is the youngest person to climb Mount Everest, the tallest mountain in the world. This mountain is just over 29,000 feet high. It's as high as almost 97 football fields.

Getting to the very top of this mountain is an amazing feat for most people, and even more amazing for a young boy. It didn't come easy. Jordan wasn't able to climb that mountain overnight. It took a lot of time, training, practice, and preparation so he could see his dream come true.

In his blog, Jordan wrote, "Every step I take is finally toward the biggest goal of my life, to stand on top of the world." Accomplishing his goal required him to take one step at a time. His dream wouldn't become a reality in the blink of an eye. It would take time.

All good things take time. It takes time for a seed to become a tree. It takes time for a puppy to become a dog. It takes time for a baby to grow up. On your journey to becoming a fit child, parent, and family, you have to remember that gaining health takes time. If you haven't been eating healthy or exercising, you can't expect to make huge changes fast. Pace yourself. Just as with making dreams come true, getting healthy will take time.

Something to Talk About

1. As a family, share some of your health goals with each other.

Maybe you, the parent, want to lose 20 pounds. Maybe you, the child, want to be more active and play sports.

2. Do you get frustrated when you want to do something, but it takes longer than you think? Such as learning to ride a bike? Or reading a book?

3. How can you be more patient with yourself and understand that sometimes you will need more time to get something done?

Tip of the Day

Instead of grabbing some chips or a candy bar as a snack, grab a piece of fruit. It'll give you energy and make you feel great.

DAY 5—WHAT DOES GOD SAY?

———————— A Word from Amy ————————

Something to Think About

If you have a dream or goal in mind, write it down. Writing down your goals will help you accomplish them.

Maybe as your mother or father is reading this today, you're thinking, *But I don't know what they are,* or *I don't think I have any.* Did you know that God cares about you so much that He has placed special desires in your heart that are unique to you? That's right! Psalm 37:4 tells us, "Delight yourself in the LORD and he will give you the desires of your heart." Well, He knows all about your heart because He created you. And because He created you, it means He created those desires too.

Ask God what His purpose is for your life. You should pray as a family, but also take some time and pray on your own. It doesn't have to be a long prayer and you don't have to use big, fancy words. Just spend time with God and ask Him.

Something to Talk About

1. How does it feel knowing that God cares about your dreams?

2. Is there something you think He may want you to do? Do you feel a tug on your heart to do something specific?

3. Spend some time speaking into each other's life. Tell each member of your family something you think they are really good at.

Tip of the Day

Go through a magazine and find a picture of something or someone who inspires you. It could be an athlete, a doctor, or a youth leader because those are things you may want to do when you grow up. Paste it on the refrigerator so you can be inspired to dream.

DAY 6—IT TAKES FAITH

A Word from Amy

Something to Think About

The Bible tells us that "faith is being sure of what we hope for and certain of what we do not see" (Hebrews 11:1). Do you understand what that means? I admit I was confused about this verse for a long time.

One pastor explained that the faith in your heart is like a blueprint for what you hope for. It's a plan that shows what something will look like after it's made. If you draw up a blueprint for a car, for example, the blueprint is not the actual car. It's proof that you are planning to build a car, and when you are done building it, that's what it will look like.

So what exactly is faith? Faith believes without a shadow of doubt that the dream in your heart will happen. You may have been too afraid to believe big things for your life. You may have tried and failed before. You may have been disappointed by other people letting you down. Let me encourage you today to never give up the faith.

Keep the faith. Why? Because dreaming takes faith. You can't dream if you don't have faith. Maybe today you need a faith boost. Maybe you feel tired or sick or afraid or don't believe that God has something special in store for you and that He will give you everything you need for your dream to become real.

Something to Talk About

1. What does faith mean to you? Is it something you don't understand yet? Is it something that you only hear your Sunday school teacher talk about?

2. What are some things that you have faith in? For instance, do you have faith that your mom and dad will shelter, clothe, and feed you? Do you have faith that God will take care of you?

3. The Bible tells us that "with God all things are possible" (Matthew 19:26). Do you believe this? Why or why not?

Tip of the Day

Are fruits and vegetables too expensive to buy at the store? Check to see if any local farms in your area sell produce.

DAY 7—DREAMS AND CHALLENGES

——— A Word from Amy ———

Something to Think About

Life comes with challenges. Bob Wieland is less than 3 feet tall, but his spirit is 300 feet tall. Bob lost both legs in a war that happened many years ago. When he returned home after his injury, he was sad for a long time.

Here's the good news. Bob didn't let his injury stop him from living out his dreams. In time, Bob completed a couple of marathons (26-mile races), was named the "Most Courageous Man in America," and even became the strength and motivation coach for the Green Bay Packers football team. What's even more remarkable is his biggest success. Bob actually walked across the entire United States...on his hands. That's right! He attached some leather shoes to his hands and pushed himself forward, step by step, with his arms.

It took him a long time, but Bob accomplished his goal. It took him three years, eight months, and six days. He walked an average of three to five miles a day. Bob's message is simple: Despite the obstacles and challenges life may present, you can always find a way to win.

Don't let your dreams die because getting there might get tough. Don't stop believing in yourself when you are tired or weak. Keep going. Keep believing. Keep dreaming.

Something to Talk About

1. How does Bob's story inspire you?

2. What are some things you are having a rough time with while you dream big for yourself?

3. How can you encourage one another as a family when the going gets tough?

Tip of the Day

Praying together is a great way to encourage one another in life, especially as we look to the future with our dreams. Take a few minutes today and pray for one another about specific needs each person may have that may be preventing them from realizing their dreams.

DAY 8—GOD'S DREAMERS

—————————— A Word from Amy ——————————

Something to Think About

When you are dreaming big things for your life, you might find that some people around you aren't as excited as you are. They may say discouraging things like, "Who do you think you are?" or "Are you sure you really want to do this?" or "You're wasting your time."

One of our favorite Bible characters is Joseph. Some of you may remember him as having a coat of many colors (as in the Broadway play *Joseph and the Amazing Technicolor Dreamcoat*). Joseph was a dreamer. He also had a lot of brothers who hated him for it. See, God gave Joseph a special gift of having dreams that meant something in real life. And they were dreams about Joseph having authority over his brothers. Every time he had a dream and shared it with his brothers, they would get upset at him. They were really jealous of Joseph, and one day they took their jealousy too far. Joseph's brothers sold him as a slave and lied to their father about it.

Years later, even as a slave and in prison, God used Joseph and his gift of dreams, and eventually Joseph became the second-in-command of Egypt. Even though this young man had to go through a lot of hardship, he never stopped dreaming. And even though his life probably looked different from what he imagined, God still used his dreams.

Don't let others discourage you from your dreams. Don't listen to people who tell you that you are not good enough. Always remember that God believes in you!

Something to Talk About

1. Are some people in your life discouraging you from your dreams? What can you do to not be influenced by their negative words?

2. Who are two or three people in your life who believe in you? Make it a point to tell them how much you appreciate their encouragement.

3. As a family, how can you encourage one another to go after your dreams and to pursue a healthy lifestyle?

Tip of the Day

Don't eat in front of the TV. Eat at the kitchen or dining-room table so you can take your time and really enjoy what you are eating.

DAY 9—GOD'S TEMPLE

A Word from Amy

Something to Think About

Have you ever had to save up your money to buy a toy or video game you really wanted? Maybe you had to cut grass or babysit, but whatever you did took a lot of work to buy that prized possession. When you bought it, I bet you took really good care of it. I bet you made sure that your brother didn't get his hands on it and break it. I bet if it was a video game, you always stored it in its case so it wouldn't get scratched. You cherished that item because it was valuable to you.

Did you know that you are God's prized possession? Did you know that He paid the highest price ever for *you*? He gave His only Son to die on the cross so He could hang out and have a relationship with you. God has big plans for your life, and *you* are what He dreams about. How cool is that?

Since you are so precious to God, shouldn't you take really good care of yourself? The Bible actually says that your body is a temple or house of the Holy Spirit. Not the church building you go to, but your body! You want God's house to be healthy, right? God has big dreams for you, so remember that when it comes to taking care of your temple.

Something to Talk About

1. What are some ways you can take better care of your temple?

2. Why do you think that you matter to God? What price did He pay for you?

3. Name some things that you cherish. How do you treat or take care of those things?

Tip of the Day

Look under your bed and see if you have stuffed any junk under there. Take a few minutes to clean and organize that stuff. When you have less clutter, it helps you to feel better.

DAY 10—YOU ARE A GIFT

Something to Think About

Have you ever been given a present for your birthday or Christmas that was wrapped so pretty you couldn't wait to see what was inside? Maybe when no one was looking, you shook it a few times to figure out what it was.

Guess what? You are one of God's presents to the world. There are gifts inside of you that only you have. You are unique and special, and your dreams are the clues to what is inside God's "present." What do I mean by that? When you dream about something you want to do or be when you grow up, it's as though you are shaking that wrapped gift. Your dreams are the clues to the plan God has for your life.

What are your clues? Do you dream about traveling to other countries? Do you dream about flying an airplane? Do you dream about being a mom or dad? Whatever your dreams are, they are a part of what makes you *you*. They are your desires, and the Bible says that God gives us the desires of our heart (see Psalm 37:4). When we realize that some dreams are given to us by God, we can use them to help guide our future.

I'm sure that your dreams include being healthy and happy. That's why it's so important to start now and make your health a priority. No one wants to open a present that has been broken. Make sure you don't let anything come between you being the best present you can be.

Something to Talk About

1. How can what you dream about hold a clue to your future?

2. What do you want to be when you grow up? How could being unhealthy prevent you from doing that?

3. Why do you need to be healthy to live out your dreams?

Tip of the Day

Make a "Life List" of things you want to do in your life. If you want to go to Europe or climb Mount Rainer, write it down. If you write down your goals, you'll be more likely to try to achieve them and mark them off the list.

Face the Facts

G ood health is a big deal. When we are healthy, we have more energy. We are more fit. We have less of a chance of getting sick or getting diseases. And being healthy means we generally feel better inside and out. Some days can feel like a chore when it comes to focusing on your health, but through these challenges, you'll learn more about why you need to keep going and not quit.

DAY 11—THE IMPORTANCE OF BEING HEALTHY

A Word from Amy

Something to Think About

When I tried losing weight before the show, I didn't do it for the right reasons. I just wanted to wear pretty clothes and look skinny. What I didn't know about being overweight was all the bad stuff that was happening inside my body where I couldn't see it.

I went to a doctor one day and he took a picture of my insides. I was shocked at what I saw. The extra fat was not only showing on the outside, but it was right there on the inside, crowding around my organs and keeping them from working properly. My lungs had so much fat around them I couldn't breathe well. This is why I got out of breath so quickly when I would try to run. The extra fat was also crowding around my heart, intestines, and stomach. All these organs need to work properly for you to be healthy and feel well.

It's fun to think about looking good on the outside, but what we need to focus on is our insides. Remember, you are valuable and need to be healthy to fulfill your purpose in life. Take care of your insides and the outside will follow.

Something to Talk About

1. Why should we think about more than just our outward appearance when it comes to our health?

2. Do you have any physical symptoms that might indicate you are unhealthy in some area? Do you get out of breath easily or do you get tired during the day at school?

3. Name three things you can do to keep your insides healthy.

Tip of the Day

Cardio exercise—such as running, swimming, and playing sports like basketball and soccer—is good for your heart and lungs. Try to do some type of physical activity five days a week.

DAY 12—"NO" MAY MEAN "I LOVE YOU"

A Word from Amy

Something to Think About

Can you remember a time that you really, really wanted something and your mom or dad told you no? Chances are, you were pretty upset. You may have even had a little pity party, stuck your lip out, or slammed a door or two.

When you don't get what you ask for, it can make you sad or even mad sometimes. That's a normal reaction. But here's the scoop. When your parents say no, it's usually because they love you and are trying to protect you.

For instance, your mom might say no at the grocery store when you beg her to buy you cookies or your dad tells you no when you beg for candy at the checkout lane. Even though it doesn't feel like it at the time, by saying no, your parents are taking care of your health.

Did you know that because sugar is high in calories, too much sugar in your diet can be a contributing factor in a disease called diabetes? Diabetes is a condition where the body can't process sugar properly. Sometimes people who have diabetes have to take insulin shots every day to make them feel better. You wouldn't want to have to do that, would you? So the next time your mom or dad says no when you ask them for a sugary snack or drink, remember that they are really saying, "I love you."

Something to Talk About

1. Discuss a time or two when your parents told you no.

2. How did it make you feel? Mom or Dad, explain to your child your reason for saying no.

3. Why is eating too much sugar bad?

Tip of the Day

Type 2 diabetes is a disease that affects more and more children. Do some research as a family about this condition so you can understand it better.

DAY 13—MY FEET ARE KILLING ME!

A Word from Amy

Something to Think About

Most of us know that when we are overweight, it makes us feel bad physically; we usually feel tired and sluggish. We also know how bad it is for our heart, lungs, and other organs. What we don't think about very often is how extra weight is especially hard on our feet.

Our feet are amazing little machines, but God built them to carry only so much weight. When we carry extra weight on our bodies, especially when we are young, it can cause us to have problems with our feet. We may get flat feet, a condition where our feet have little to no arch in them. Having flat feet can lead to an overload on our joints and tendons. This can cause our feet and legs to be in pain all the time. When we are in pain, the last thing we want to do is exercise. When we don't exercise, we become inactive and lazy. See how this vicious circle can hold you back from being healthy?

What can you do to change this? You can make sure you maintain a healthy weight or lose weight if you need to. You also need to make sure that you are wearing proper shoes so that your feet get the right support they need. A good pair of running shoes will fix this problem.

So pay attention to your feet and take care of them. They are the only ones you have!

Something to Talk About

1. Why is it so important to your feet that you maintain a healthy weight?

2. What can happen to your body if you carry an excessive amount of weight?

3. What are some ways you can take care of your feet?

Tip of the Day

Try to buy your shoes at a store that caters to runners and other athletes. The people who work there can help you determine the type of shoe that's best for you.

DAY 14—A MATTER OF THE HEART

A Word from Amy

Something to Think About

I recently met a young man who weighed over 400 pounds. He knew he needed to change his life and was making plans to work on his weight. He was funny, sweet, and full of life. He was the kind of guy you would want to be friends with. Three weeks later I got a message from his brother telling me that this young man had died from an enlarged heart.

I was shocked by the news. Although I know that we need to take care of our health so we can live a long life, I had never been touched by the reality of it in this way. This guy was so young and would have had his whole life ahead of him had he started taking care of his health as a child. He will never have the chance to live out his dreams. It's a great loss.

When we eat the wrong foods, don't get any exercise, or carry too much weight on our body, it puts stress on our heart. We can start now to make sure we protect our heart by eating right and exercising regularly. We need to keep our heart healthy. It truly is a matter of life or death.

Something to Talk About

1. What are some ways to keep your heart healthy?

2. Do you have any people in your life who have or had heart problems?

3. Exercise plays a big part in protecting your heart. Discuss some active things you can do as a family that will help keep your heart healthy.

Tip of the Day

Jumping rope is a great cardiovascular exercise. Have a jump-rope competition as a family. See which member has the most consecutive jumps. The winner gets to choose what you have for dinner. (Make sure it's healthy!)

DAY 15—RUN YOUR RACE

--------------------------- A Word from Amy ---------------------------

Something to Think About

Have you ever challenged your sister or brother to a race? When you were running, I bet you didn't carry a heavy toy or put on your heaviest coat. I'm sure you had on your best running shoes and you threw off your coat or sweatshirt so nothing would hold you back. You couldn't afford to have extra weight slow you down. You wanted to win!

Did you know we are running a spiritual race? The Bible says in Hebrews 12:1 (NLT), "Therefore, since we are surrounded by such a huge crowd of witnesses to the life of faith, let us strip off every weight that slows us down, especially the sin that so easily trips us up. And let us run with endurance the race God has set before us."

What does that mean? I believe some things can hold us back from living the life God wants us to live. Eating junk food and not getting enough exercise could be some of them. So can being disobedient to our parents or mean to someone in our class. We must lay those things aside because those weights can hold us back from winning in life. Just as you wouldn't run a race carrying something heavy, you don't want anything to prevent you from living your best life.

Sometimes our bad choices, bad habits, or bad attitudes can be like weights. Don't let bad choices, habits, or attitudes negatively influence your life. Get rid of them!

Something to Talk About

1. What kinds of choices can you make that can help you run a good race in life?

2. What kind of choices have you made that are not so good?

3. How can those bad choices weigh you down when you're running your spiritual race?

Tip of the Day

Run a race in the yard with your friends. Try it first carrying something heavy and have your parents record your time. Then run it again without the weights and see how much faster you can run!

DAY 16—THE HEAVY BOOK BAG

—————————— A Word from Amy ——————————

Something to Think About

Have you ever had to carry your book bag when it was full of all your books and papers? Maybe you had a lot of homework that day and had to stuff it to the max and carry it home from school. I bet it sure was heavy. Maybe so heavy that it made your back and shoulders hurt. What a relief when you finally got to take it off!

Now imagine if you had that much extra weight on your body all the time. It would be hard to run around and play. It might even make you tired, cranky, sluggish, or sick. This is why we need to watch the foods we eat and keep our body active. If we just lie around on the sofa, watch television, and eat potato chips all day, before we know it we can put on extra weight (just like stuffing our book bag full). But unlike the book bag, which we can take off instantly, it's much harder to take extra weight off of our bodies.

Extra weight puts pressure on your lungs so it becomes harder to breathe. It puts pressure on your knees and joints so they hurt more. And it makes you tired. Who wants to feel all that? So think about how heavy that book bag feels when you're carrying it, and let it remind you to keep your body healthy.

Something to Talk About

1. How does it feel when you have to carry around a heavy weight?

2. Name a few things that carrying extra weight can do to your body.

3. What types of activities do you like to do that having extra weight could prevent you from doing as well?

Tip of the Day

Stuff your book bag full of heavy books. Put it on your back and walk around the house for an hour and see how it makes you feel.

DAY 17—CHART YOUR COURSE

—————————— A Note from Phil ——————————

Something to Think About

Have you ever pretended you were a great explorer who was going to travel to faraway places? If you did, the first thing you might have done was gather some friends to go with you and look at a map (even if you drew it yourself) to plan the route you were going to take. You probably described to them the treacherous terrain, vicious animals, and evil villains you might encounter along the way. I'm sure you also bagged a lunch and some supplies to take on your journey.

Did you know that life is really a big adventure? It's full of wonder and possibilities and good things that you can do and see. But you have to be prepared. You have to chart your course to help guard against pitfalls that can come. Some of those pitfalls can include eating too many sugary snacks and drinking too much soda. They can make your blood sugar drop and can make you really cranky. They can also be a factor in developing type 2 diabetes, which you know is a serious disease.

Think of poor health as an evil villain you can defeat on your journey by eating more fruit for snacks and drinking water rather than sodas. You don't want to get defeated on your journey, so chart your course for success!

Something to Talk About

1. What are some things you can do on your journey to make sure your future is healthy?

2. Name some foods that can contribute to diabetes and heart disease. What are some foods that are good for you?

3. Why is taking care of your health one of the things you need to have on your map for your life?

Tip of the Day

Help your mom pack a healthy picnic basket or your lunch bag for school. Talk about which foods are healthy choices and which foods are unhealthy choices.

DAY 18—BE A WINNER

A Note from Phil

Something to Think About

Don't you love it when football season comes around? I sure do. I love the chill in the air that signals the beginning of fall, the energy of the crowd in the stadium, and watching the players run down the field in their new uniforms. You can feel the excitement in the air as people cheer for their favorite team to score the touchdown or kick the field goal that wins the game.

It must be really cool to be one of those players on game day and have everyone cheering for you. But in order to play in the game, those players first have to train. Did you know that football players train really hard for many hours a day to get ready for a big game? They run sprints, they lift weights, they participate in drills, and they practice again and again the plays they're going to use in the game. It's hard work!

In order to be a winner, you have to train for it. In order to be an athlete, you need to be willing to do the work. In order to be healthy, you have to focus on the things you can do to be healthy. Often it's not easy, but hard work and training are the difference between being average and being a winner.

The road to good health may be hard sometimes, but don't give up. Stick it out so you can be a winner!

Something to Talk About

1. Have you ever played a sport where you had to practice really hard? What kind of things helped you be a better player?

2. In what ways can you train to be a winner in your health?

3. What types of activities can you do that will help make you strong?

Tip of the Day

Go outside and throw the football around with your parents. It's good exercise and a whole lot of fun.

DAY 19—SINGING THE BLUES

———————— A Word from Amy ————————

Something to Think About

Some days you just get up on the wrong side of the bed. Do you know what I'm talking about? It's the kind of day when it seems as though nothing is going the way you want it to go, and it makes you feel pretty bummed out. Everyone has blue days every now and then. This is normal when it happens occasionally. But if you're feeling low a lot, then the culprit might be what you're eating. It's true! Food can affect your mood more than you may realize.

Let's pretend you're a car. In order for a car to run, it has to have gas, right? Well, our bodies are similar. We have to put the right food in our "tanks" so that we run properly. If we don't eat foods that are nutritionally balanced, it's like putting the wrong kind of gas in your car. It will drive sluggish and slow.

Why does this happen? Because our bodies need the proper nutrition to keep our blood sugar stable. Have you ever eaten candy or cookies and for a little while you had a whole bunch of energy? Then before you knew it, you got really tired and cranky. This happens because sweets raise our blood-sugar level for a short time, but then it drops.

We can keep this crazy ride from happening by eating meals that are good for us and that include a combination of protein, carbohydrates, and a little healthy fat. Keep this in mind when you put "gas" in your tank, and it will help you fight the blues.

Something to Talk About

1. Talk about some foods that you like. Which category do they fall into: protein, carbs, or fat? See how many balanced combinations you can come up with.

2. What does your blood sugar have to do with your mood?

3. Think about times when you felt sad or down. Could they have had something to do with something you ate?

Tip of the Day

Prove the blood-sugar theory. Next time you eat a bag of candy or some other sugary treat, pay close attention to your emotions. Do you feel the roller-coaster high and then sudden low?

DAY 20—DEFEATING THE LAZY MONSTER

A Word from Amy

Something to Think About

If you are like many kids (including mine), I bet you love to play video games. It's fun to play in another world and become a different person. Some of my kids' favorite games are the kind where they defeat a bad guy and become the hero who saves the day. Who doesn't want to defeat bad guys?

Well, did you know there's a bad guy who wants to take over your life and make your body unhealthy? I like to call him the "Lazy Monster." The Lazy Monster comes around and whispers in your ear, "Why don't you lie on the sofa and watch TV? It's so comfy!" or "You can play outside when you get to the next level on your video game." The Lazy Monster's main goal is to keep you from being active. He wants you to be lazy and unhealthy.

But you can be the hero and defeat the Lazy Monster! How can you do this? You can choose to be active and play outside instead. You can call your friends and go ride your bikes. You can play basketball and other sports. If you defeat the Lazy Monster, you can also defeat his partners in crime—the Diabetes Dude, the Heartbreaker, and Mr. Grumpy. These cohorts are very dangerous to your health. They love for you to be lazy because then they will be in control and defeat you.

Don't let them do that. Get active and be your body's hero!

Something to Talk About

1. What are some ways that you can defeat the Lazy Monster?

2. Why should you move your body?

3. How can you bring activity into your life every day?

Tip of the Day

Play a game of HORSE on the basketball court with your parents, siblings, or friends. It's a fun way to be active and defeat the Lazy Monster.

Your Kids Are Watching You

You can't expect your kids to magically pick up a healthy lifestyle if you are not riding the same train. Your children look up to you and pay attention to what you do, say, and think. Get inspired to set the example in your household. Eat better. Be more active. And see the possibilities that open up once you begin to lead your family into better health.

DAY 21—BEING ACCOUNTABLE

Something to Think About

One of the first things we did when we were chosen for *The Biggest Loser* was to get on the scale and show millions of Americans how much we weighed. You can imagine how embarrassing that was because we were so fat! But it was a big part of making a change in my life. I knew I couldn't hide that I needed to lose weight. I needed to be accountable for my health. "Being accountable" means taking responsibility for your health. It also might involve letting someone know of your struggle and asking them to help you change.

Maybe you don't need to lose weight, but you feel as though you would die if you had to stop drinking soda, enjoying a dessert after each meal, or eating ice cream every day. When food has this kind of power over you, it can destroy your health. You must be accountable to your parents (and parents, you can be accountable to other people in your life) and let them know that you need their help to change your bad habits.

As you go through these challenges, I encourage you to be honest. Be an open book. If you have a problem, admit it. Maybe you can't stop eating in the middle of the night. Or maybe you can't stop playing video games. Whatever your area of struggle, share it with someone so they can help you find a solution. The Bible tells us to confess our faults to one another so that we may be healed (James 5:16).

Don't be afraid to tell the truth; it brings freedom.

Something to Talk About

1. What are some things that may have power over you?
2. Who can you talk to regularly who will hold you accountable for your actions?
3. What does the Bible say to do so that you "may be healed"?

Tip of the Day

Try giving up something that you love for one week. If you have a hard time doing this, it probably has more power over you than it should.

DAY 22—CHOICES

A Word from Amy

Something to Think About

The Bible says that the nation of Israel was given the choice between life and death, a blessing and a curse (Deuteronomy 11:26). What does that mean for us? Like the people of Israel, we can make good choices or bad ones. We can make healthy choices or unhealthy ones. If you think about it, every time we make a choice that is good for our body, we are making a statement that we are choosing life.

I don't always make the right choice. I have been known to mess up sometimes. And I can't blame anyone else when I don't do the right thing because I made the decision. I can't blame my mom, dad, sister, brother, or friends when I don't eat right, exercise, or drink water. When it's all said and done, the only one who has the power to change and make good choices is me. The ability to choose is so powerful. We are ultimately the one in control of what we choose to do with our lives.

When we choose to eat healthy and be more active, we are making the choice to have a healthier life. Our parents can't make the choice for us because we have been given that responsibility.

So tell yourself who's the boss (you are!). Make the right choices and choose life. And parents, make sure you make good decisions before you tell your children to make them. Practice what you preach.

Something to Talk About

1. Who has the power to make choices in your life?

2. What are some good choices you make every day?

3. Can you blame your parents, teachers, or friends when you make bad choices that have bad results?

Tip of the Day

When you buy a snack, make sure you read the label on the package. The label will guide you as to whether it is a healthy choice.

DAY 23—ATTITUDE

A Word from Amy

Something to Think About

Has your mom or dad ever told you that you needed an attitude adjustment? Maybe they said it when you were grumpy or disobedient. Do you know that you have the power to decide whether you're going to have a good or bad attitude? You can choose whether you look at things positively or negatively.

If you see a glass filled halfway with water, do you view the glass as half-full or half-empty? Your outlook holds a clue to your attitude. I love the saying that life is 10 percent what happens to us and 90 percent how we respond to it. We may not be able to always change the world we see around us, but we can change the way we see the world.

My son Rhett, who is autistic, is one of my heroes. All of his classmates and teachers can tell you that there is rarely a day where he is not the happiest and most excited person in the room. He wakes up early every day, even on Saturday, with a big smile on his face. I watch him and sometimes wonder what it must be like to be so carefree. To watch the joy he has for the simple things in life is no less than a gift.

Our attitude truly makes all the difference. In this journey to get fit and healthy, make sure you keep a good attitude. If you do, you are guaranteed to be more successful. You can do it. I know you can. And parents, guide your kids in having a positive attitude. You are their best teacher.

Something to Talk About

1. Why should we keep a good attitude?

2. What are some "attitude adjustments" you might need to make?

3. How can your attitude make a difference in your journey to get healthy?

Tip of the Day

Counting your blessings is a great way to change your attitude from negative to positive. You might even want to make a list of all the blessings in your life.

DAY 24—IF IT DOESN'T WORK, FIX IT!

A Word from Amy

Something to Think About

One of the definitions of insanity is doing the same thing over and over and expecting a different result. Have you ever played basketball and found yourself shooting the ball the same way over and over? Even though you didn't make a basket the first five times, you expected it somehow to go in on your sixth attempt.

Good health doesn't come by continuing to do the same old things that don't work. You have to make changes that cause you to be healthy. You can't eat pizza, candy, and chips every day and not expect to eventually pay for it with your health. Mark my words, you will have to pay for your bad choices. If you want things to be better, you have to decide to make them better.

Good health begins with the "want" to change. Then you need to take the steps to improve your life. If you're not being as active as you need to be, get moving. If you're eating too much junk food, eat natural foods instead. I spent many years making wrong choices, but once I decided to make the change, I knew I had to learn from my mistakes and do better. I had to come to the point where I wanted to change, and I had to do it for myself.

It takes desire, courage, and strength to start walking somewhere you have never been before. The journey toward health begins with you realizing you have to take the first step. Mom or Dad, I challenge you to take that first step so you can lead your child in taking her first step.

Something to Talk About

1. What is the first step in making a change?

2. How might mistakes become valuable teaching tools?

3. What is the definition of insanity cited in today's reading?

Tip of the Day

Think about the seasons of the year and how they change. Think about how people grow and change. Write down a few changes that you have experienced in your life and changes that you would like to see happen.

DAY 25—BEFORE THE DAWN

A Word from Amy

Something to Think About

Can you remember a time when you just didn't want to do something? I know I can. I had the hardest time getting out of bed this morning at 5:00 for my daily run. I just didn't want to do it. It was way too early. Then when I went outside, I thought it was too cold. Then as I started to run, all I could think about was how hard it was to breathe. Then my leg started to hurt. Everything was bothering me, and my body and mind were trying to get me to stop. But I knew I had to do it, and just like the Energizer Bunny, I kept going and going and going. And I ended up having one of the longest and best runs I've had in a while.

As I was getting close to the end of my run, the song "Yahweh" by U2 came on my iPod. The song talks about how pain precedes the birth of a child. In other words, there is always struggle before a great victory. When I heard that song, I felt the runner's high. It gave me the strength to push myself to finish my run. Endorphins and good feelings washed over me, and I felt a sense of accomplishment.

Why do we have to struggle to succeed? I don't know. But I do know that it is always the darkest before dawn. The breakthrough will come if you don't quit. Keep going toward your goals. Don't ever give up and quit.

Something to Talk About

1. Was there ever a time you forced yourself to do something and afterwards felt great about it?

2. What are some challenges that can make you stronger?

3. Why should we never quit when challenges come?

Tip of the Day

Try running really fast for 10 minutes. It will probably be hard while you're doing it, but just wait and see how great you feel when you're finished.

DAY 26—BREAKING FREE

———————————— A Word from Amy ————————————

Something to Think About

Yesterday I was walking through my house, and suddenly I remembered what it felt like to be a prisoner in my own body. Because I've been on my journey to better health for a long time, it's easy to forget the desperation I used to feel. I used to be so tired when my children asked me to do something. Finding the motivation to go anywhere (even to the mall) was a challenge. One of the biggest motivators and joys for me is to remember what a great feeling it is to be free from poor health, excess weight, and unhealthy habits.

You are in the process of making a prison break. You have already come so far, and I am so very proud of you. I encourage you to keep up the good work and to keep going. Remember, every day that you choose to exercise and eat healthy, you are chipping away at the chains of poor health, bit by bit.

You are a beautiful, valuable creation of God. You are made in His image. He has a plan for your life that is far above what you have for it. I challenge you today to dream bigger, reach higher, and break free of those chains.

Something to Talk About

1. What are some things you can do to break out of the prison of unhealthy habits?

2. What are some prisons that people create for themselves with bad habits?

3. How can you break free from any bad habits you might have?

Tip of the Day

Have you ever seen Chinese handcuffs? They are little stretchy tubes you put on your fingers, and when you pull against them they get tighter. It's only when you relax that they come right off. Try relaxing a little today and let the cares of the day fall off of you.

DAY 27—CLEAN YOUR ROOM

—————————— A Word from Amy ——————————

Something to Think About

Have you ever had a chore to do, such as cleaning your room, that you kept putting off? Maybe you started to do it, but the room was so dirty that you shoved everything under the bed and told yourself you would clean it tomorrow. And maybe it's still dirty because the job seems so big that you are too overwhelmed to start.

Sometimes doing our homework, cleaning out a room in our house, or even getting healthier seems so hard that we keep pushing them to the bottom of our to-do list. We find other things to do instead. Wouldn't it be better just to go ahead and do those things so they don't bother us every day? Of course it would.

So where do you start? First, make a mental decision that you are going to do something about it. You may not feel like it, but your mind is stronger than your feelings. Your mind tells you what to do. Second, break down the project into manageable steps. I heard someone once say, "How do you eat an elephant? One bite at a time." Taking small steps is what gets a big job done.

So no more shoving things in your life under the bed. Face whatever you need to face and just get it done.

Something to Talk About

1. What is something that seems so overwhelming that you keep putting it off?

2. What are some strategies you can use to make the job more manageable?

3. Why is getting healthy like cleaning your room?

Tip of the Day

When you're cleaning your room, throw or give away everything that you haven't used in the past six months. If you have gone that long without using it, you probably don't need it cluttering up your room.

DAY 28—IT'S TIME TO PRUNE

—————————— A Word from Amy ——————————

Something to Think About

Don't you just love the spring? The whole world comes alive after a long, cold winter. Did you know that in order for those trees and flowers to bloom so beautifully, the dead stalks and branches have to be trimmed back? This is called pruning.

In the same sense, we have to prune some things from our lives in order to reach our full potential. Jesus tells us in John 15:2 that He prunes every branch that bears fruit so it can bear even more fruit. This is also similar to the law of sowing and reaping. If you do good things, you will get good things; if you do bad things, you will get bad things.

Being on this "Challenge" is the perfect time to get rid of some bad things that may keep you from finishing strong. You may need to prune friends who don't support you or who keep you from your health goals. You may need to prune activities, such as watching too much TV, that take up a lot of time. You may need to prune bad habits from your life. If you are anything like me, maybe you rely on food to comfort you in times of depression and stress. You will need to let go of these habits and replace them with better ones, such as eating healthy snacks, relaxing in a long bath, or going to the gym.

Pruning is not easy and it can be painful. Always keep the goal in mind. Pruning is necessary to make room for the new you. So let go of anything today that might be holding you back.

Something to Talk About

1. Why might you need to prune some things from your life?

2. Can you identify anything you need to prune?

3. What does the Bible say about pruning?

Tip of the Day

Start a savings account and put money in it every week. See how fast the law of sowing and reaping works in growing your money.

DAY 29—PEARL OF GREAT PRICE

A Word from Amy

Something to Think About

What things do you place the most value on? What means more to you than anything in the world? I'm sure you would list your family, friends, and your relationship with God. But what else is valuable? A special toy? A favorite game?

I've been thinking about that a lot lately. There are things we should value above all else and things we should place little value on. It's never a bad idea to look at our priorities and see if there are places where we might be a little unbalanced.

Having good relationships with our family is important. Doing well in school is important. Having fun with our friends is important. But we also need to put our attention on being healthy. None of the things we value mean anything if we aren't healthy enough to enjoy them.

I love the parable in the Bible about a man who heard about an extraordinary pearl. It meant so much to him that he sold all he had to buy this treasure. It was the most valuable thing he had ever seen in his life. It meant enough to him that he sacrificed everything for it. My health is that pearl for me. It is worth sacrificing time and money for it.

What about you? Will you value your health so much that you're willing to sacrifice some things that are standing in your way? Will you take the time to exercise for at least a little while every day? Will you be careful about what you eat so that you can keep your body strong? You have only one body and one life to live, so take care of it.

Something to Talk About

1. What are some things that are valuable to you?

2. What would you be willing to sacrifice in order to acquire good health?

3. Why should you manage your time well when it comes to making your health a priority?

Tip of the Day

Make a list of the most important people and things in your life. Where does health show up on the list?

DAY 30—ELIMINATING THE EXCUSES

A Word from Amy

Something to Think About

A college professor of mine once said that the definition of an excuse was "a skin of a reason stuffed with a lie." I always thought that was a mean thing to say (probably because I always had an excuse for why I couldn't get my homework in on time). The truth is, we lie to ourselves a lot because we think we have good reasons not to change.

How many times have you waited until the last minute to complete a homework assignment or a project? And how many times could you not finish it on time? Did you have an excuse ready to give your teacher?

We can always find a reason why we couldn't do something we were supposed to do.

We do the same thing with our health. We make excuses about why we ate too much and didn't exercise enough. There is always a party to go to, a movie to watch, or a vacation to go on where we have a "reason" to give ourselves a break. The problem is that we will never change for the better if we keep making excuses for our bad choices.

When we got the call to be on *The Biggest Loser,* we moved heaven and earth in a week so that we would be able to go. We did whatever we had to do because we knew we were doing it for our health. If you want to change your life, you have to do what you need to do and eliminate the excuses.

Don't let excuses hold you back from living the best and longest life you can. Don't say, "I can't do this because..." To borrow a phrase from Nike—Just do it.

Something to Talk About

1. What are some excuses you have made in the past?

2. What is the definition of an excuse that my professor gave me?

3. Why are excuses bad?

Tip of the Day

If you are constantly late, try setting your clocks 10 minutes early. That way if you are always 10 minutes late, at least you'll be on time.

Nutrition Sense
for Your Family

It's time to learn how and what to eat. Proper nutrition is a big part of what it means to be healthy, so pay close attention. You'll learn about why you should eat natural foods such as grains, fruits, and vegetables and drink lots of water. And you will understand that feeding your body well helps to keep it running properly, just as putting the right fuel in your gas tank makes your car run like it should.

DAY 31—GROW YOUR OWN VEGGIES!

A Word from Amy

Something to Think About

What do you think about when I say the words "the great outdoors"? Do you think about breathing in fresh air? The smell of freshly cut grass? There's nothing quite like spending time outside. It makes you feel so good.

The outdoors is also where food grows. Not only that, you can even grow your own food. Back in the old days, there was no such thing as grocery stores. Most families grew their own fruits, vegetables, and grains.

Imagine planting a seed in the ground, watering it, fertilizing it, and after a couple weeks, seeing that tiny seed sprout into a tomato plant that eventually produces tomatoes you can hold in your hand. How awesome is that!

Take a family trip to a local gardening store and talk to someone about building your own garden. Start out with veggies that are easy to grow, such as tomatoes, green beans, carrots, and beets. Add different food items to your garden every year. If you live in an area where you can't grow a garden, visit a local farm that allows you to pick your own fruits and vegetables. It'll be a fun family day out, and you can learn how food grows.

Above all else—and I know many of you have heard it said a thousand times before—eat your veggies. Try to eat two cups of veggies a day. They're good for you.

Something to Talk About

1. What are your favorite veggies?

2. Why are veggies good for you?

3. Here is another fun project to do as a family. The next time you go grocery shopping, spend some extra time in the produce section. Go through each section and check out the different kinds of cool looking vegetables. Hold a big red beet in your hand. Check out the unique shape of an eggplant and its deep purple color. Try a new veggie every week.

Tip of the Day

To help your child make healthier food choices, make a daily vegetable and fruit chart and post it on your refrigerator. Have your child color a picture or place a sticker or gold star for each fruit or vegetable eaten.

DAY 32—SAY "NO" TO THE DRIVE-THRU

———————————— A Note from Phil ————————————

Something to Think About

I hate to break it to you, but fast food is not a part of a nutritious diet. Most foods that you get at the drive-thru window are loaded with extra junk to make the food taste better, but it's bad for your body.

I know we live in a busy time and sometimes it's just easier to grab lunch or dinner on the road when you're on your way to soccer practice or a play date. But while it's easier, is it good for you? Absolutely not.

In their excellent book *Chew on This,* Eric Schlosser and Charles Wilson talk about the dangers of fast food. They say, "The food you eat enters your body and literally becomes a part of you. It helps determine whether you'll be short or tall, weak or strong, thin or fat. It helps determine whether you will enjoy a long, healthy life or die young."

Ouch! Why eat fast food if you can eat healthier at home? You can even eat healthier on the road. Pack lunch or dinner to take with you. Take some fruit or veggie snacks to the game or on your play date. There are many ways you can be healthy even when your life is super busy. Remember, you have to fuel your body properly for it to work properly. And fast food is not the way to do it. Natural foods are the way to go.

Something to Talk About

1. Do you like fast food? Why or why not? How does it make you feel an hour or so after you eat it? Do you feel tired or energized?

2. What are some ways you can take healthy food with you when you're on the road?

3. Knowing how bad fast food is for your body, do you still want to eat it? Why or why not?

Tip of the Day

Slow down while you're eating. It takes 15 minutes for your digestive system to tell your brain that you are full. The best way to eat slower is to chew each mouthful 30 times. When you eat, take your time!

DAY 33—ENCOURAGE YOUR FRIENDS TO MAKE HEALTHY CHOICES

A Word from Amy

Something to Think About

"I'll trade you my banana for your potato chips."

"I'll give you my carrot sticks for your cupcake."

Sound familiar? Making healthy choices with your friends at school can be a hard thing to do sometimes. Especially when you sit with them at the cafeteria and see some of their lunches (that you think taste super good, but are not the best things to eat for good health).

Sometimes when you make healthy choices, your friends won't be as excited as you are. Though you may love apples, they may not be used to eating them. It's okay. Here is a great opportunity to teach your friends, by your example, how to make the right choices when it comes to nutrition.

Instead of telling someone what to do, it's better to show them by doing it yourself. This is a great reminder for parents. When you offer fruits and veggies to your kids at mealtime, make sure you eat them yourself. We make a greater difference when we lead by example.

Remember this, kids. You might need to learn how to say no more often (not to your parents, but to your friends who don't make the right nutrition choices). When they're munching away on salty or greasy foods and offer you a bite, tell them "No thanks," and munch on a piece of fruit instead. When they gulp down a ton of soda and ask if you want a Coke, say "No thanks," and drink your water instead.

Something to Talk About

1. How many of your friends make healthy eating choices?

2. If they eat snacks or a meal that's not the best choice to fuel their body, do you feel pressure to do the same thing?

3. How can you encourage your friends to make the right nutrition choices?

Tip of the Day

I know you probably hear it all the time, but take care of your teeth. Brush them at least twice a day. When you eat foods that are high in sugar (candy or soda) or starches (french fries or cookies), it can cause tooth decay. Good nutrition even matters in keeping your beautiful smile.

DAY 34—WHAT DO YOU SEE?

—————————— A Note from Phil ——————————

Something to Think About

Have you ever looked at a special image where there's a picture hidden inside a picture? You have to stare at it long and hard until you see something that pops out. You are surprised when you see it, but it was there all along. Then when you look at that secret image any time afterward, it is as clear as day.

I want to show you something you may have looked at hundreds of times before, but may have missed. When you cut open a tomato, the inside is red and has four chambers. Our heart also is red and has four chambers. Tomatoes have this thing called *lycopene* in them. Lycopene is a great tool to help maintain good heart health. As a matter of fact, all fruits, vegetables, and beans have nutrients in them that help your body, and many of them resemble a part of your body.

Celery, bok choy, and rhubarb look like and are helpful to your bones. Kidney beans help maintain kidney function, and yes, they are shaped like a kidney. When cracked open, walnuts, which help our brain function, look like the human brain. Grapes hang in a cluster that has a shape similar to that of the heart; each grape looks like a blood cell. Research shows that grapes are a heart and blood-vitalizing food. Onions, which look like your blood cells, have been shown to help clear waste materials from blood cells.

The next time you eat your fruits and veggies, think about how God designed each of these foods to help your body.

Something to Talk About

1. What vegetables help the blood cells?

2. What organ do kidney beans help?

3. What do celery, bok choy, and rhubarb help?

Tip of the Day

What kind of fruit do you like? When you're tempted to eat junk food, pick up a piece of your favorite fruit instead.

DAY 35—AN APPLE A DAY KEEPS THE DOCTOR AWAY

———————— A Word from Amy ————————

Something to Think About

Does an apple a day really keep the doctor away? Maybe. Did you know an apple provides nine of the sixteen chemical elements and four of the six most crucial vitamins required by our body to function and protect itself against disease? But an apple is just one of the many fruits God made to keep us healthy.

Fruit is a carbohydrate and carbohydrates give us energy for our day. We always try to mix a carb with a protein to keep our blood sugar stable. For example, when you're eating an apple or orange, have some nuts or cheese with it. If you're having Greek yogurt, put some peaches or berries in it. One of my favorite snacks is a banana with a little peanut butter.

How much fruit should we eat? Nutritionists suggest two to four servings a day. There are so many delicious ways to get your daily amount of fruit. I usually eat fruit for my snacks, or I put it in my cereal or oatmeal for breakfast. You can have your mom or dad pack a piece in your lunch box or you can eat one after school for a snack. I like to freeze grapes and pop them in my mouth like candy. You can also blend frozen fruit (such as strawberries) and a bit of milk to make a sorbet or a smoothie.

Fruit is a wonderful source of vitamins, fiber, and antioxidants. It is nature's dessert and it is yummy.

Something to Talk About

1. What are some things that fruit does for our bodies?

2. What should you eat with fruit?

3. What are some ways to put more fruit into your diet?

Tip of the Day

Put snacks in little plastic bags. Measure them out in single-serving portions so you eat only as much as you are supposed to.

DAY 36—ARE YOUR EYES BIGGER THAN YOUR STOMACH?

—— A Word from Amy ——

Something to Think About

Have you ever noticed that when you stub your toe, you immediately feel pain? The same is true when you skin your knee. Your brain will quickly send a message to your nerves to tell your body that you've injured yourself.

This isn't true when it comes to eating and feeling full. We can eat a giant meal and not feel full immediately. It takes the brain longer to send the message to our stomach that it needs to stop eating. We need to know the right portions. We can't count on our stomachs to tell us.

Here are some helpful hints:

- one serving of fruit/vegetables = a balled-up fist
- one serving of meats/protein (and take the fatty skin off) = a deck of cards
- one serving of bread/grains/pasta = a tennis ball
- one serving of dairy such as cheese (choose the low-fat kind) = the size of four small dice
- one serving of oil/fats/sweets = one teaspoon or the size of a small die

Cup your hands together and hold them out. That's roughly the size of your stomach. Can you imagine how much we stretch our stomachs when we eat a hamburger, fries, and a chocolate milk shake?

Here's a key to remember. If you are super tired after eating, you probably ate too much. Food should energize you, not make you want to take a nap. Stick with eating small portions more often (instead of three huge meals a day), and you'll be headed on the right track to good health.

Something to Talk About

1. What is the right portion for a single serving of protein? How about oils, fats, and sweets?
2. What does it mean if you are tired after a meal?
3. How big is your stomach?

Tip of the Day

Have a deck of cards, a tennis ball, and some dice handy in your kitchen so you can compare them to the amount of food you put on your plate. You will soon notice that you are eating much less.

DAY 37—FAT BROTHERS

—————————— A Word from Amy ——————————

Something to Think About

Imagine you are friends with two brothers. They live in the same house and have the same last name, but one is bad news while the other is a really great guy. This is the case with the "fat brothers," saturated and unsaturated fat.

Saturated fat is the bad news brother. He can be found hiding in candy, cookies, cakes, pies, chocolate, french fries, and other things that are bad for you. What happens when you have too much saturated fat in your diet? It forces your body to create more cholesterol. When the levels of cholesterol in your blood are too high, you put yourself at risk for all kinds of diseases.

The good brother is unsaturated fat. He's a great friend of your body because he helps burn extra body fat. Eating good unsaturated fats in foods such as olive oil, nuts, and nut butters keeps your hunger under control, and these fats also produce hormones that help your muscles grow. Good fat also does something else. It helps deliver vitamins A, D, E, and K to your fatty tissue to be used when your liver needs them.

Fat has a bad reputation, but it's only saturated fat that you need to quit hanging out with. Become friends with unsaturated fat, and he will help you be healthier.

Something to Talk About

1. What is the difference between saturated and unsaturated fat?
2. What foods have saturated fat in them? What foods have unsaturated fat in them?
3. What good things can unsaturated fat do for your body?

Tip of the Day

Look in your pantry and fridge and read the labels on some of your foods. Do you see any with a lot of the "bad brother" in them? Stay away from these foods.

DAY 38—SUGAR AND SPICE IS NOT SO NICE

Something to Think About

Do you remember the nursery rhyme that said that little girls were made of sugar and spice and everything nice? Well, it turns out that too much sugar and the spice salt are not so nice to your body. They are things you want to watch out for if you want to stay healthy.

Sugar is everywhere. It's found in soda, condiments, cereals, and even places you wouldn't expect it, like some yogurts and bread. Sugar is dangerous because it is nutritionally empty. It doesn't fuel your body as other foods do. It also causes your blood sugar to spike up and then crash back down. This is why when you drink a soda, you feel a rush of energy, but later you feel sleepy or cranky. Too much sugar also puts you at risk for obesity and type 2 diabetes. We need to be careful that we eat sugar only in very small amounts to keep our body working well.

We also have to be careful about eating too much salt. It can make you retain fluid, contribute to high blood pressure, and overwork the kidneys and liver. We get plenty of salt in our regular foods, so it's not necessary to add salt to the food on our plate. Instead of salt, many other spices can be used to give your food flavor.

Watch out for sugar and salt in your food because they are not very nice to your body. Too much of them does more harm than good.

Something to Talk About

1. Do you like to eat foods that are high in sugar or salt?

2. What foods are high in sugar? Salt?

3. What are some of the health problems that may occur if you consume too much sugar and salt?

Tip of the Day

Next time you're in the grocery store, take a trip down the aisle with the spices and seasonings. Pick out a few that you would like to try on your food.

DAY 39—THE THREE AMIGOS

A Word from Amy

Something to Think About

Ever notice how some things take more than one person to do them? For example, it would be really hard to ride on a seesaw or play baseball by yourself, right? The same thing is true when it comes to fueling your body. One type of food can't do the job alone.

Three macronutrients are needed to run your body well. I like to call them the "three amigos" of nutrition. They are protein, complex carbohydrates, and healthy fat. Each of these macronutrients is like a piece of a puzzle needed to make a healthy meal. Each of them has a specific job to do to make your body run at its best.

Protein repairs your muscle and helps it recover from exertion, and is found in such foods as lean meat, turkey, fish, chicken, eggs, skim milk, low-fat cheese, and cottage cheese. Carbohydrates give you energy and help your brain function properly. Complex carbohydrates come from fruits, vegetables, brown rice, whole-wheat bread, wheat pasta, quinoa, and sweet potatoes. Fat has the job of keeping your cells healthy. Your hair, nails, and skin are healthier when you have a little healthy fat in your diet. Some good sources of healthy fats are peanut butter, almonds, walnuts, olive oil, and sunflower seeds.

When the three amigos are together on your plate, they give you energy and keep your blood sugar stable so you don't feel tired all the time. When your body is working properly, you feel better. Get healthy and start making friends with the three amigos.

Something to Talk About

1. What are the three amigos of nutrition?
2. What does protein do for your body?
3. Why should we combine these three "friends" at every meal and snack?

Tip of the Day

Work with your mom and dad to plan meals that combine protein, complex carbohydrates, and healthy fat.

DAY 40—DRINK UP!

A Word from Amy

Something to Think About

We cannot live without water. God created our body to be made of over 50 percent water. Here are some reasons that water helps us (and why we should drink lots of it every day):

- It flushes out toxins (chemicals and poisons that aren't good for us).
- It keeps our body temperature and metabolic rate normal.
- It helps our organs to work properly.
- It aids the production of enzymes that help us digest our food.
- It maintains healthy skin and hair.
- It helps our body absorb essential vitamins and minerals.

Water also keeps us hydrated. Over 50 percent of Americans are dehydrated. Here's how you can tell if you're dehydrated. (I'll warn you, though, it may be kind of gross.) The next time you go to the bathroom, check out the color of your urine. If it's pale yellow or clear, you're probably hydrated (good job!). If it's a deep yellow color, you need to be drinking more water. Here's a tip. Don't wait until you're thirsty. Drink water all day. When you're thirsty, it's too late. You're probably already dehydrated.

Have your mom or dad pack a water bottle in your lunch box so you can keep filling it up at school. If you go for a walk, a bike ride, or play a sport, always have water with you. Did you also know that sodas actually make you thirstier? Water is the only thing that can truly quench your thirst. So don't forget to drink your water.

Something to Talk About

1. What are two reasons you should drink water?
2. What are some ways you can make sure to drink more water?
3. What color should your urine be if you are hydrated?

Tip of the Day

Do what the doctors recommend: Drink eight glasses or more of water every day.

Activate Your Kids

Fitness can be fun. It can be a time where you bond with your kids, get your heart pumping, and enjoy some laughs. Don't think of fitness as a chore or something you *have* to do. Think of it as giving your body boosts of energy with activities that are fun. In this section, you'll learn about all sorts of cool things to do that will make you feel good inside and out.

A Word from Amy

Something to Think About

I got my first bike on my seventh birthday. My mom and dad took me to Sears to pick out the one I wanted. It was pink with a white basket covered with multicolored plastic flowers. When my dad finished putting it together, I jumped on it and rode up and down the driveway all day until it got dark. My mom had to make me come in!

That summer I spent almost every day riding around the neighborhood on my bike. I fell off many times and have many scars to prove it. But I never stopped riding. At that time, there were no video games to play and no cable television to watch. It was just me and my bike, the great outdoors, and the wind in my face.

When I got older, my cousin and I rode our bikes to the nearby woods and made our very own secret clubhouse. On one of our bike journeys, we discovered a creek and built a mini dam and pond. We felt like Robinson Crusoe with our own little world. We didn't need television to tell us about adventures because we were making our own.

Maybe you've never had the wonderful feeling of exploring and having adventures on your bike. If not, I challenge you to put down the video controller and the TV remote for one week and do something outdoors. If you don't have a bike, you could ride a scooter, skateboard, or get on some inline skates. There's a whole world out there waiting for you to explore.

Something to Talk About

1. What adventures could you have if you played outside more?

2. Why should you get out into the great outdoors instead of staying inside all the time?

3. How do you think that staying outside more could be helpful to your health?

Tip of the Day

Plan an adventure outdoors in your neighborhood today. Pack a lunch and plenty of water, grab a friend or family member, and go see how many new places you can find.

DAY 42—THINK TO WIN

Something to Think About

I don't know when, but somewhere along the way, I formed an opinion about myself. It could have been the time I tried out for basketball in junior high and didn't make the team. Or the time I joined a new gym and the trainer worked me so hard that I was throwing up before the session was over. Whenever it was, I had lived all my life thinking that I was not a winner. I didn't think I could excel at any sport because I was never good enough. Though I had a good attitude, I never excelled physically.

I found I was limiting myself with this attitude. Why can't you have both? Why can't you have the best attitude and be the best on the team? I'm here to tell you that if you believe you can, then you can!

When I started working on my health and working out a lot, I realized that I was competitive. I loved a challenge. I loved to work hard and I loved to win. I didn't let my old mentality stop me from enjoying success at whatever I was doing. I believed I was a winner, and I was going to prove it.

Don't let a self-defeating attitude stop you from becoming good at a sport. Don't allow negative thoughts, such as *I'm playing just to have fun* or *I'm just the nice person on the team*, keep you from being the best. Play with all your heart and see yourself as a winner.

Something to Talk About

1. Has a certain thought ever kept you from getting fit?

2. Can you be a good sport and a good athlete?

3. What can you tell yourself to make you work harder at a sport?

Tip of the Day

Listen to your coaches and parents. They have lived longer and have more experience than you do. If you listen to what they tell you to do, you may learn something.

DAY 43—FIELD DAY

—————————————— A Word from Amy ——————————————

Something to Think About

On the last day of spring term, my school held an annual event called "Field Day." The students were always gushing with excitement when this day came. On Field Day, each class competed against the other classes in such games as the sack race, the three-legged race, tug-of-war, and the egg toss. The winners would get blue ribbons, and the rest of the kids would get ribbons of other colors. It was so much fun, but it was also a chance to exercise. At the end of the day, we students were tired but happy after being active and competitive.

What if your family organized your own Field Day right in your backyard? Wouldn't that be a great way to get active and help you be healthier? You can do a three-legged race. You can do an egg toss. You can play tug-of-war. And you can play all these games using common household items.

Today, plan a Field Day for your family. Encourage your friends or neighbors to join in the fun. Everyone will have a great time and have an opportunity to activate their body.

Something to Talk About

1. What are some other games you can come up with for your Field Day?

2. What items do you have in your house that can be used for these games?

3. How can Field Day activities help make you fit?

Tip of the Day

Go to the dollar store and buy cheap ribbons or prizes you can use to reward the winners of your Field Day games. It will inspire friendly competition.

DAY 44—IT'S THE CLIMB

A Word from Amy

Something to Think About

The first challenge I had on *The Biggest Loser* was to climb a steep hill behind the ranch. The trail was a mile long, up and back. Before then, I hardly ever climbed the stairs in my own home, so you can imagine how overwhelming the task was. It was far more exercise than I was used to.

I remember that day well. It was hot, and we contestants were sweaty and thirsty. As we walked, we found it hard to breathe and our legs really hurt. But we kept walking until we reached the summit. Once we got there, we looked around us, and my breath was taken away. A beautiful valley down below stretched as far as my eye could see.

We immediately forgot about the struggle to get up there because the picturesque setting was incredible. At that moment, I realized I had been limiting my life. I spent most of my days sitting on the sofa and not moving my body, when I could have been visiting places like that mountain and enjoying the beauty that God has created for our enjoyment.

Can you relate? Have you been keeping your sofa warm and missing out on all those places you could be exploring? I'm sure you know Miley Cyrus's song "The Climb." It talks about how life is like climbing a mountain and the moments in life that you remember are in the challenges you face. If you never get off the sofa, then you really aren't living your life. So get up and get active and take the climb to enjoy a little beauty.

Something to Talk About

1. What are some things you haven't been able to enjoy because you haven't been active?

2. In what way is mountain climbing good for your body?

3. Why is climbing a mountain a lot like facing life's challenges?

Tip of the Day

Before you spend a day outdoors doing any vigorous exercise, make sure you eat a healthy meal loaded with complex carbohydrates for energy.

DAY 45—P.E. IS FUN

—————————— A Word from Amy ——————————

Something to Think About

When I was in elementary school, I loved gym class. We did such fun things as square dancing, kite flying, and bowling. Of course we also played the standard games of kickball and softball and had fitness tests, but our teacher always made sure we had fun. She understood that we could get physical activity from all kinds of movement, not just the traditional ways.

When I got to middle school, it was a different story. Gym class was about being competitive, and because I was overweight and had low self-esteem, I felt as if I couldn't compete. I wasn't as good as the other kids. I couldn't run as fast or throw a ball as far, so I got easily discouraged. I dreaded class and couldn't wait for it to be over. Gym wasn't fun anymore.

How about you? Do you hate going to gym class or do you look forward to it? If you've started believing, for whatever reason, that gym isn't fun, you may have built up a wall in your mind. I encourage you today to break down that wall. Go to class and give it your best shot. If you put your heart into it, you'll do great, and you'll have fun in the process.

Something to Talk About

1. How can your attitude make gym more fun?

2. What are some fun things you do in gym class?

3. If there are activities in class you don't enjoy, explain why you feel that way.

Tip of the Day

Always go to gym class prepared. Make sure you have an extra pair of socks, your gym uniform, and tennis shoes.

DAY 46—RUNNING YOUR RACE

A Word from Amy

Something to Think About

When I was a little kid, my sisters and I would have races in our backyard. I loved the feeling of running with the wind blowing through my hair. I also loved to win (and since I was the oldest, I won most of the races!). Now that I'm older, I still like to run in races. I'm not trying to win first place, but I run my best. And I love the feeling I get when I cross the finish line. I know that I've accomplished something many other people haven't.

If you haven't signed up for a race, I want to motivate you to go for it. People of all ages run, and they are usually doing it to support a worthy cause. Gather together your parents, siblings, and even your grandparents to run. It's a fun family activity, and running is great exercise for your heart and lungs.

I ran my first 10-kilometer race (10K) in New York. At one point, I ran over the George Washington Bridge. It was amazing to run over that great landmark. It was also a great feeling knowing I was doing something that was benefiting my body and my mind. When I crossed the finish line, people were cheering for us and handing out bottles of water. I felt so proud.

I want you to have that same feeling, so make up your mind to run a race. Most of them are advertised online, so go on the Web and see what's offered in your area.

Something to Talk About

1. In what ways is running good for your body?
2. What is a good reason to run a race?
3. How can you find out if there are any races in your area?

Tip of the Day

When running a race, make sure you pace yourself. You don't want to run really fast at first and use up all your energy before you reach the finish line. Take your time and have fun.

DAY 47—MIX-UP THE CARDIO

——————————— A Word from Amy ———————————

Something to Think About

If you've already started activating your body, you probably noticed you have a lot more energy than when you started. Now I want you to push yourself a little harder. You always want to challenge yourself, because once your body gets used to a certain level of effort, your fitness progress slows down. Also, if you are anything like me, you probably get bored easily. Sometimes just walking every day for a month doesn't cut it. You want to be constantly looking for different types of cardio exercises that are fun.

There are a bunch of cardio options to choose from. Some you may not be able to do well in the beginning, but after a couple of times, you will build up your stamina and your muscles. Here are some activities you can try to get your body moving:

- running up stadium bleachers
- swimming
- exercise DVDs
- dancing
- football
- racquetball
- basketball
- tennis
- baseball/softball
- boxing
- stair-climber
- stationary bike
- hiking
- gymnastics
- karate
- soccer
- kickball
- cycling
- chores such as raking leaves, moving furniture, and cleaning your room (your parents will love that one!)

Open yourself up to the exercise possibilities and keep that body moving.

Something to Talk About

1. Look at the list above and pick three activities you would like to try.

2. What are some other activities you can think of to get cardio exercise?

3. Why do you want to continue to push yourself when it comes to exercising?

Tip of the Day

Jumping on a trampoline is great exercise. If you have one, jump on it for 15 minutes and see how much fun it is.

DAY 48—PLAY YOUR GAME

A Word from Amy

Something to Think About

When my kids were little, I signed them up for all kinds of sports. We tried soccer, basketball, and baseball, to name a few. Baseball didn't work because my oldest son played outfield, and he wouldn't pay attention and would never notice when the ball came his way. In soccer, my kids were known for running the wrong way. Basketball wasn't good either. They got tired of running up and down the court and would just stop in the middle of the game.

After some time, I let them choose the sport they wanted to try. One of my sons tried skateboarding, and it helped him with his balance, agility, strength, and confidence. Another son tried cross-country running. He loved it. It took some time, but eventually they all found a sport they liked and were really good at.

Playing sports is a fun way to exercise. It's good for your development and growth, and it builds confidence. Maybe you've had a hard time finding a sport you can play well. You may have thought you weren't athletic because the sports you tried weren't right for you. I encourage you today to keep trying new sports. Eventually, just like our boys, you'll find what works for you.

Remember, it doesn't have to be a traditional team sport such as football, baseball, basketball, or soccer. It could be swimming, various Frisbee games, beach volleyball, running, cycling, tennis, golf, surfing, or skateboarding. Keep trying new things and play your game.

Something to Talk About

1. What kind of nontraditional sports do you like to do?

2. Why is it a good idea to play sports?

3. What are some sports that you have tried that weren't a good fit? What did you not like about them?

Tip of the Day

Whatever sport you play, make sure to always wear the proper protective gear. Helmets when you are cycling and skateboarding are a must.

DAY 49—TAKE A HIKE

A Word from Amy

Something to Think About

Don't you just love to spend time outdoors? I do. One of the coolest ways to get exercise and also spend time together with your family is to go for a hike. What's more fun than hiking up a mountain and getting to be in the middle of God's creation?

Hiking is good cardiovascular exercise because it gets your heart rate up. It's also a great way to strengthen your leg muscles because some hikes require you to walk on a steep incline. The neat thing about hiking is that you can get so wrapped up in the beautiful nature and scenery that it doesn't seem like hard work. Exercise is great when it doesn't feel like exercise.

Our family has hiked in Paris Mountain State Park several times. The park has many beautiful trails that run along shallow creeks and ponds. When you get to the top of the mountain, the view is extraordinary. You feel like a pioneer on an adventure. It's a great feeling to share with your family.

We don't have to always think of exercise as something competitive or difficult. Exercise can come in the form of a peaceful mountain trail on a warm summer day. So go ahead, take a hike.

Something to Talk About

1. What are some ways that hiking helps your body?

2. Why is hiking a good family activity?

3. Does exercise always have to be competitive?

Tip of the Day

When you go hiking, make sure to bring plenty of water and some snacks. You can make your own trail mix using almonds, granola, and dried cranberries.

DAY 50—YOUR OBSTACLE COURSE

———————— A Word from Amy ————————

Something to Think About

Phillip and I did something really fun last year. We participated in an obstacle course called the "Mud Run." The first thing we had to do was dive into a pit of muddy water and swim through it under a net. Then we had to crawl under a military Hummer, scale high walls, wade through creeks, swing on ropes, and finally, we had to run four miles. While we were competing, we felt like soldiers in a jungle. Let me tell you, it was tough! There were some moments where I wondered, *What have I gotten myself into?* It was a dirty, sweaty, and fun event, and when I finished, I felt great.

That obstacle course is a lot like life. At times it's challenging and you just want to quit. That's when you need to dig down and find the resolve to keep moving. The same thing is true for your journey to be healthy. Sure, it may be easier to sit on the sofa or play video games all day instead of playing a sport or taking a hike. But you won't succeed on the path to good health if you don't push through the hard times and get active.

Today, get out there and move your body. Be the master of your obstacle course.

Something to Talk About

1. What kind of obstacles do you need to overcome when it comes to your health?

2. What are some mental obstacles that you face when it comes to exercise?

3. Why does it make you feel good to overcome challenges?

Tip of the Day

Organize your own neighborhood obstacle course. Use your play set, sprinklers, water slides, old tires, or anything that can make it challenging.

Finding Balance

Life usually doesn't go according to our plans or schedules. And while it's necessary to maintain a healthy lifestyle to live an optimal life, it can get challenging sometimes. Especially when we get detoured along our journey by things out of our control. Learn how to find balance just when you need it most so you don't get off track on your journey to good health.

DAY 51—**BALANCING ACT**

Something to Think About

Have you ever been to the circus and seen the seal that balances on a ball and also balances a ball on its nose? Do you ever feel like that seal? Having to balance school, homework, sports, friends, and your chores? You may feel that if you add one more thing to your life, you'll fall off the ball. Well, sometimes you have to fall off the ball and mix things up a little to actually make changes that are good for your life. There are times when we have to be a little out of balance in order to put our focus on a particular goal.

If you were driving a car and it started sliding toward the ditch, you would have to jerk the steering wheel to get the car back where it's supposed to be. For a minute, everything might feel chaotic, but it's necessary to get the car back in the right place.

It's the same thing with our health. At first it may seem that the changes you're making are actually making life harder, but in the long run it will be worth it. When I was gaining health, the majority of my focus was on losing weight and exercising more. I rearranged my whole life to meet that goal. I realized that in order for me to be successful, I had to focus completely on what I wanted to achieve.

Give yourself permission to focus on being the best you can be. Balance will come back to your life in time.

Something to Talk About

1. In what ways is it good to have a little chaos in your life?
2. What things can you stop doing so much so you can focus on the goal of being healthier? Watching too much TV? Playing video games?
3. Do you ever feel as if you have a lot to do but not enough time?

Tip of the Day

If you don't have one already, get a day planner and get organized. Effective time management is a big key to creating balance.

DAY 52—FEAR FACTOR

Something to Think About

Have you ever wondered why so many times in the Bible God tells someone to "fear not"? Do you think maybe it's because He knew what a big deal that message is and that we would always need to be reminded of it?

Fear is everywhere. If you watch the news, there is always something to be afraid of—cancer and other diseases, car accidents, violent crimes, deadly earthquakes, a bad economy. I don't watch the news anymore because I don't want to be frightened by the negative and scary information being reported.

Let's be honest. There are a lot of things we can be afraid of, but fear is not the only thing out there. We also have hope. The best part of trusting in God is that we can believe that everything will work out the way it's supposed to. The Bible tells us that "the LORD directs the steps of the godly" (Psalm 37:23 NLT). This verse has given me much comfort over the years through my own trials. If I trust God and do the right thing, then He will direct my path. Through Him, I will fulfill my purpose and destiny. This verse gives me the permission to mentally relax.

Any fear you have will only hold you back. It's time to let go of fear and trust God with your life while you are on your path to getting healthy.

Something to Talk About

1. Read Psalm 37:23 in the Bible. What does it mean to you?

2. What are some of your fears?

3. What should you do when you're afraid?

Tip of the Day

Every time you think of something that scares you, pray. Ask God to help you trust Him more than your fears.

DAY 53—**PERSEVERANCE**

A Word from Amy

Something to Think About

Ever have one of those days when nothing goes right? Of course you have. Everybody does. It's a part of life. During those times, it's easy to get discouraged and think you're never going to reach your goals. This is when you have to persevere, which is a big word for "stick it out and don't quit."

In my journey to get healthy, there were times that I wanted to give up. Maybe you have felt the same way. So what can we do when we're tempted to quit? The short answer is: the right thing. We will all have days when we're tired, sick, unmotivated, or just don't want to eat healthy and be active. Those are the days when you cannot quit. You have to keep going.

This is true for anything that truly matters in life. The winner is often the one who perseveres. Winners know if they will not quit, they will win. Think about all the people who have started something great and quit. They might have had a bad day or series of bad days and just gave up on their dreams. They may have stopped short of doing something great because they didn't persevere. I cannot begin to tell you how many times during my journey that my mind told me I was not going to make it. But I refused to give up and kept going. And guess what? I made it. And you can too.

Life will always have its ups and downs. But never let the downs stop you from moving forward.

Something to Talk About

1. What is something that winners know?

2. What does *perseverance* mean?

3. Have you ever felt like quitting? What did you do?

Tip of the Day

Running up bleacher stairs is one way you can get some good cardio exercise. Check with a local high school to see if they will let you use the bleachers at their football field. Then see how many times you can run up and down them and test your limits.

DAY 54—LIFE ON THE EDGE

A Word from Amy

Something to Think About

How many of us dream about having a normal (which to most of us means boring) life? Very few of us, I'm sure. When I was a little girl, I wanted to be a country-music singer. Almost every day, I would stand in the living room and sing at the top of my lungs. My dad was a radio announcer, and for my sixth birthday, he surprised me by taking me to a country-music show where I met a famous country singer. I even got to sit on her lap while she was waiting to go on stage. I was so happy, I felt as if I were in a movie.

Unfortunately, I couldn't sing very well, so I let go of that dream. My point is, no one ever says, "I want to be ordinary when I grow up." We all start out dreaming big dreams such as wanting to be an astronaut, a doctor, or even the president of the United States. We all want to live a life that's on the edge and that contributes to mankind in a significant way.

I'm convinced that we allow setbacks in life to keep us from dreaming. When we experience heartbreak or difficulty, we want to protect ourselves from feeling pain again. But to live a balanced and healthy life, you have to dream. Do the hard work and challenge yourself, but never forget the importance of dreaming.

If you get knocked down, get back up. If you fail, try again. If life throws you a curveball, keep swinging the bat. If we keep focused on being great in whatever we do, we will always live a life on the edge.

Something to Talk About

1. What do you want to be when you grow up?

2. What do you do when life throws you a curveball?

3. What do we allow to cause us to stop dreaming?

Tip of the Day

Make a list of what you think is great about you. See how many things you can write down, and ask your friends and family to add to it.

DAY 55—**MIDDLE OF THE ROAD**

—————————————— A Word from Amy ——————————————

Something to Think About

My oldest son just got his learner's permit to drive. His dad is too afraid to take him driving, so I've been chosen as his "instructor." I've noticed on these scary (for me, at least) drives that he tends to go too far over on the right side of the road. He focuses on the oncoming cars so much that it makes him veer toward the opposite side of the road. I find myself constantly telling him to drive closer to the middle.

It's the same in our lives. We can get so excited about something that we focus only on that one thing. Before we know it, everything else gets ignored. For example, we can put so much attention on our friends that we neglect our schoolwork or we can put so much time into having fun that we neglect our responsibilities at home.

We can't be extreme in any area because that takes us out of balance. Think about this. No one wants to sit in a chair that has one leg longer than the others; it's crooked and hard to stay on. When we are out of balance, we become like that unstable chair. We need to keep all our legs, all our activities, in balance.

Something to Talk About

1. What are some areas in your life that you tend to focus on more than others?

2. What happens when we focus on only one thing?

3. Why is balance important?

Tip of the Day

Here's a great way to get organized. Buy a family calendar where you can write down all the activities and events that family members are involved in. Use different color markers for each person.

DAY 56—**SNOW DAY**

—————————————— A Word from Amy ——————————————

Something to Think About

Where I live in the South, it doesn't snow very often. When it does, it's such a rare event that everything shuts down. This is a beautiful time where my little corner of the world gets covered in a white blanket and my family gets to snuggle up in the house together. We love to watch old movies in front of a fire and drink hot chocolate and eat popcorn.

On days like these, I've always felt that I had permission to be a little lazy. I can relax and not think about any work or responsibilities because God is giving me the day off. All of us appreciate this day of rest.

Just like your family, ours can get a little busy with school, after-school activities, and church events. Sometimes we have so much going on that it's easy to get burned out. To have a balanced life, we need to make sure that we take time to enjoy ourselves and relax.

It's not good to sit in front of the television all the time, but it's good to have a family movie night or game night once a week. It's not good to ignore your responsibilities, but it's always a good idea to go on family vacations or even spend a day doing something fun.

All work and no play makes life dull. Don't forget to take time to enjoy life and each other.

Something to Talk About

1. What are some things you like to do as a family to relax?

2. Do you get snow days? Does your family do anything special on those days?

3. What is your dream vacation?

Tip of the Day

Make a "family fun night" jar. Get some note cards and have everyone write down something fun they would like to do as a family. Put the cards in the jar, and once a week, pull one out and do it.

DAY 57—RIDING THE ROLLER COASTER

A Word from Amy

Something to Think About

Isn't it fun to ride on a roller coaster? The anticipation you feel when you slowly go up the incline and then the thrill of the sudden drop is both scary and exciting. Riding a real roller coaster is fun, but it's not fun when you're riding one with your energy levels. I'm talking about being up one minute and down the next. One minute you feel happy and full of energy, and the next you are tired and cranky.

You ride the energy roller coaster because your body isn't getting the proper fuel it needs, and your blood sugar gets out of balance. When you are unbalanced, your energy levels go out of whack. The only way to keep it balanced is to eat whole, healthy foods and to always combine a protein with a carbohydrate.

We need to eat the right stuff. Sugary foods such as candy, cookies, and sodas are an instant ticket on the energy roller coaster. The sugar quickly gets into your bloodstream and gives you a sugar high for a while, and then it takes you back down the hill.

Remember, keeping balance in your life starts with what you eat. So choose your food wisely and keep off the roller coaster.

Something to Talk About

1. What foods are an instant ticket on the energy roller coaster?
2. What should you always eat together to keep your blood sugar stable?
3. How do you feel when your blood sugar is not stable?

Tip of the Day

Part of keeping your blood sugar stable starts with eating a balanced breakfast. Stay away from sugary cereals and choose a whole-grain cereal and some form of protein, such as eggs or turkey bacon or sausage.

DAY 58—SUPPORT: EVERYONE NEEDS IT

--------- A Word from Amy ---------

Something to Think About

I can't tell you the exact day it happened, but I remember one day thinking about my life and realizing that I had a lot of people around me helping me get healthy. I had a doctor, a dietician, a therapist, my family, and my friends to support and encourage me. I was also fortunate to have an amazing trainer and coach when I first lost a lot of weight. He would pick me up on Saturdays, and we would hike or run bleachers at the local high school. He held me accountable each and every day. I truly believe I would not be where I am today without his encouragement.

I want you to remember one thing: Everyone needs a coach. A coach challenges and pushes you. A coach will help you realize your potential. I have friends who are very successful, and every time they take on a new project, they hire a coach. This is the strategy of many wealthy and successful people. Even famous athletes have coaches. A coach can be a teacher, a mentor, or even a big brother or sister who is your cheerleader during your journey to better health.

Who are the coaches in your life? Your parents, pastor, friends, or other family members? Lean on them for support, and you will be more successful in whatever you do.

Something to Talk About

1. Do you have coaches in your life?

2. What have you learned from them?

3. Why should you have support as you change your lifestyle habits for the better?

Tip of the Day

The next time you go to a sporting event, watch how the players interact with their coaches. Notice that the team looks to their coach for guidance on how to play the game and win.

—————————— A Word from Amy ——————————

Something to Think About

God made our body to need times of rest in order for us to grow strong and healthy. Your parents know this. That's why they always make sure you get enough sleep. We need eight hours of sleep per night (more if you are young) so that we can regenerate ourselves and be ready to go the next day.

Have you ever had a sleepover where you stayed up all night with your friends? Did you notice how you felt the next day? I bet you were so tired you couldn't think clearly. You probably didn't make much sense when you talked because your brain and mouth didn't seem to be working together. And I bet you went home and slept, and when you woke up, you felt like a different person.

Getting your rest is a big deal, so go to sleep and have sweet dreams about being healthy.

Something to Talk About

1. Why do we need sleep in order to be healthy?

2. How many hours of sleep do you need per night?

3. If you are not getting enough sleep, what changes do you need to make to ensure you get enough?

Tip of the Day

Make sure you try to keep a set bedtime every night. Doing that will help you get the proper amount of rest you need.

DAY 60—THE BEST MEDICINE

A Word from Amy

Something to Think About

Have you ever heard a joke or watched a funny movie that made you laugh so hard you could hardly catch your breath? Even though you couldn't breathe for a second, I bet that afterward you felt so good.

Do you know that laughing is actually good for your health? You've probably heard the saying "Laughter is the best medicine." Well, it's true. People who laugh a lot are healthier than people who are sad, mean, or angry all the time. This is just one reason why we need to make the effort to have a good time and enjoy our friends, family, and our lives.

The Bible even says in Proverbs 17:22 that "a cheerful heart is good medicine." What does it mean to have a "cheerful heart"? It means to be happy and full of joy. It's easy to get angry when someone is mean to us or upset when things don't go our way, but we should not let those feelings stay in our hearts.

If we become angry with someone, we need to forgive them quickly. When we are mad at people and don't forgive, we can get a root of bitterness in our hearts. This keeps us from being cheerful. This is not healthy for our attitude or for our bodies.

I love to be happy. I love to be around people who make me laugh. I love funny movies and television shows. I love to laugh because it makes me feel good and it's good for my heart. So keep laughing and keep being healthy.

Something to Talk About

1. Why is laughter like good medicine?

2. Why should you forgive other people?

3. What is something that makes you laugh?

Tip of the Day

Watch a funny movie tonight with your family and laugh your way to good health.

Strong Mind = Strong Body

When you want to get physically stronger, you have to start with your mind. The power to succeed is found there. Learn how to be in charge of your mind and make the commitment to never give up.

DAY 61—MENTAL STRATEGIES

————————— A Word from Amy —————————

Something to Think About

The mind is the boss over the body. It is in charge. That's why before we can get our body healthy, we need to change some things in our mind. Here's the deal. The thoughts you think and the beliefs you believe will determine the direction your life takes.

I want you to use your imagination. Think about what you want your future to look like. What kinds of things are you not able to do now that you want to do? Think about what your life will look and feel like when you are able to do those things. Think about these things with the confidence that it *will* happen and imagine what that feels like.

We all have recordings in our subconscious that we have been listening to our whole lives. These recordings are of tragedies and triumphs. If our mother told us that we were a great artist when we colored her a picture in kindergarten, we probably love art. If we were told as a child that we were an athlete, we probably see ourselves that way. If we were told we were chubby, then no matter what weight we become, we may still see ourselves as chubby. We need to make new pictures and recordings so we can see ourselves differently.

See yourself as healthy and strong. See yourself as an athlete. And today, I am telling you that you are an athlete who is healthy and strong. Now believe it for yourself.

Something to Talk About

1. What are some recordings (good or bad) you have about yourself?

2. What do you imagine your future will be like? What will it feel like?

3. In what ways does the body follow the mind?

Tip of the Day

Write down your top three goals for the next year. Establish some steps that can help you get on track to make them happen.

DAY 62—**BEING A TEAM PLAYER**

—————————— A Word from Phil ——————————

Something to Think About

Have you ever heard of the Tour de France? It's a challenging, three-week-long bike race that takes place in France and nearby countries and has about 200 riders participating in it. These cyclists ride up steep mountains, over cobblestone streets, and through the countryside. It is a grueling and treacherous ride, and only the very best riders in the world are qualified to take part in it.

The competitors in this race are members of teams. The riders in each team decide which member they want to help be the winner of the race, and the team members then work together to accomplish that goal. If that person wins the race, the entire team feels as if they, too, have won, because they all worked together. It's a great picture of teamwork. Not one person can do it all on their own. They all need each other.

God wants us to live life that same way. He called us to be a part of His team where we all win together. I like to think of this in terms of being healthy. Sometimes you feel as though you are sacrificing things (like not eating certain foods or giving up watching a TV show so you can be active instead), but you have to remember that you are choosing health so your whole family can win. Be a team player and live the life of a winner.

Something to Talk About

1. What are some ways your family is working as a team during this "Challenge"?

2. What are some areas where you can show more support to another family member to help them along?

3. What are some sacrifices that you have had to make so that the other members in your family can be successful?

Tip of the Day

Get some exercise and play flag football in your backyard. Invite the neighbors to join your family and make it a team effort.

A Note from Phil

Something to Think About

I recently watched an interview with a female professional runner from Kenya. She said something that really struck me. She said you have to train hard if you want to win easy. Toby Tanser wrote a book with the same title. In *Train Hard, Win Easy: The Kenyan Way*, he shows how the best distance runners in the world work very hard in their training. There are no shortcuts to their success. They run the best and they train the best.

Many times we do not think that the little things we do to reach our goal matter, but they do. I was in a competition to lose weight, and I was changing my life at the same time. Every single day, I made decisions to work hard and train hard. Seven months later, I had dropped 151 pounds. I kept a goal and a constant vision in front of me. I pictured what it would feel like to win. Gaining my health felt great! My life hasn't been the same since.

Every day we get to choose what we will do with our day. We can do things that are good for us or bad for us. I know sometimes it's tough to push ourselves to do something we may not want to do (though it's good for us), but when we do, the payoff is worth it. Remember, train hard to win easy.

Something to Talk About

1. Can you think of a time when you had to do something really hard, but after you did it, you felt really good about yourself?

2. How hard are you working on this "Challenge" to better your health? What can you do better?

3. What are some ways you can train hard now so that you can win easy later?

Tip of the Day

Try arm wrestling your brother, sister, friend, or parent. It's a fun game, and it makes your arms stronger!

DAY 64—CHANGING YOUR EMOTIONAL RESPONSE

—————————— A Word from Amy ——————————

Something to Think About

My parents divorced when I was 10. I was very sad when I got the news. I remember my mom saying that I was the oldest, and I had a big job now because I had to help her take care of my sisters. I know that she was trying to make me feel important, but at the time all I felt was this huge burden come over me. I had to grow up at the speed of light. It was hard for me, and I began to eat to feel better.

Have you ever felt sad and so you ate something to make you forget the pain? This is an emotional response that can be bad for your health. The only time we should be eating is when we are hungry. We shouldn't eat when we're bored or sad.

If you have this unhealthy habit, every time you go to the refrigerator, ask yourself if you are hungry or if you want to eat because something is bothering you. If you're upset, go for a walk (this helps me a lot!) or talk to your parents or a close friend. Find a buddy and go to the park or ride bikes together. There are many ways you can handle how you feel besides eating something that may be bad for you. Remember, only you can break the cycle.

Something to Talk About

1. Have you ever stuffed yourself with food because you were bored or sad?

2. Is anything bothering you now? Spend some time sharing as a family and support each other.

3. How can you work together as a family to help each other change your emotional response to food?

Tip of the Day

When someone hurts you or says something mean to you, be quick to forgive. Not forgiving someone doesn't hurt them; it only hurts you.

DAY 65—**DON'T LOOK BACK**

Something to Think About

Have you ever done something that later you wished you hadn't? Maybe you got in a fight with a good friend or told your mother you cleaned your room when you really didn't. The grown-up word for when you feel bad about things you did that are wrong is *regret*.

I know that feeling pretty well. I spent many years not taking care of my body. When I finally made the decision to get healthy, I started feeling bad about letting my body get to such an unhealthy state. But you know what I realized? That looking back at the things we've done wrong will never change anything. We can't relive the past, so it's best to learn from it, make changes for the future, and move on.

Sometimes when we look with regret at the things we've done, we get so consumed with our failures that we can't move on to new victories. The Bible says in Micah 7:19 that when we ask God to forgive our sins, He casts them into the depths of the ocean. That means He doesn't even remember them. So why should we? The Bible also says that "all have sinned and fall short of the glory of God" (Romans 3:23).

See, nobody is perfect. We all make mistakes. The key is to learn from our mistakes and do better. So don't look back. Today is the day to start over. Look forward to your new healthy future.

Something to Talk About

1. Can you name something you have done that you regret?

2. How can you learn from that mistake?

3. What are some steps you should take when you do something wrong?

Tip of the Day

Think of something you have done wrong that you feel guilty about. Write it down on a piece of paper. Now tear the paper up and throw it away. This illustrates what God does with our sins when we ask Him to forgive us.

DAY 66—TALK TO YOURSELF

—————————— A Word from Amy ——————————

Something to Think About

Have you ever seen someone talking to themselves? Maybe you looked at them and thought they were crazy. I believe that talking to yourself can be a good thing once in a while. Now before you ask the men in the white coats to take me away, listen to what I'm saying.

Getting healthy can be a struggle sometimes. There are days that you would much rather eat pizza than chicken and vegetables. There are times when you know you should do something active, and all you want to do is lie on the sofa and watch television. Those are the days when talking to yourself is a good thing. Those are the days when you need to tell yourself what to do.

When I have rough days, I tell myself that I love to exercise. Just by saying that to myself, I start to believe it. When I convince myself that I'm doing something I love to do, rather than doing it because I have to do it, it makes me want to do it. I also tell myself that I will eat healthily. If I'm the one making the choice of what food to eat, and my mom and dad aren't telling me what to do, I don't mind so much.

We are in control of our mind, but sometimes we have to trick it into doing what we want it to do. That's why talking to ourselves isn't such a bad thing. Now get out there and tell yourself who's boss.

Something to Talk About

1. What are some things you can tell yourself that will help you make the right choices?

2. Who is responsible for making the right choices in your life?

3. What can you say that will trick you into making the right choices?

Tip of the Day

When you're running down the street in your neighborhood and you start to get tired, tell yourself you're just going to run to the next mailbox.

When you get to that mailbox, tell yourself you're going to run to the stop sign and so on. By tricking yourself into running these small distances, you'll find that you will run longer than you thought possible.

DAY 67—WATCH YOUR MOUTH

A Word from Amy

Something to Think About

Has your mother ever told you to "watch your mouth!"? If she has, she was probably telling you that because you said something that wasn't nice or you talked back to her. Well, I want you to watch your mouth in a different way. I want you to watch the words you say about yourself.

I'm talking about the negative things we say, such as "I can't do it" or "I'm not good enough." No matter what you're talking about, it's never a good idea to focus on the negative. We need to say positive things about ourselves.

I always hated sports and going to gym class. I would tell myself, *I'm not the athletic type* or *I'm not able to do the same exercises as the other kids.* I found out later in life that I was telling myself lies. And I also believed all those lies for many years.

We have to say positive things about ourselves because whatever we say is what we really believe. That's what the Bible tells us: "The mouth speaks what the heart is full of" (Matthew 12:34). The truth about us is found in that great book. The Bible says such things as, "Be strong in the Lord and in his mighty power" (Ephesians 6:10), and "I can do all this through [Christ] who gives me strength" (Philippians 4:13). This is what we need to be saying about ourselves because this is the truth.

So the next time you are tempted to say something negative about yourself, don't do it. Say something positive instead.

Something to Talk About

1. What are some good things you can say about yourself?

187

2. Why is it important that we don't say negative things about ourselves?

3. What does the Bible say is the source of the words that come out of our mouth?

Tip of the Day

Put a rubber band around your wrist. Every time you catch yourself saying something negative, pull the rubber band back and give yourself a "pop." Soon you will stop yourself before you say anything negative.

DAY 68—MOVE THOSE OBSTACLES

—————————— A Word from Amy ——————————

Something to Think About

This morning I decided to get up at 5:30 and go to the gym. I was in a hurry, and the coffee I desperately needed to wake me up spilled all over my car. I didn't have enough time to eat breakfast, so my stomach was growling relentlessly. My gas tank was running on empty, so I had to stop for fuel. When I finally got to the gym, I learned the class I wanted to take wasn't scheduled until the next day. How frustrating! What do you think I did? Maybe the better question is, what would you have done in this situation?

It's easy to look at obstacles as a sign that we should just give up. But that's the opposite of what we should do! Let me tell you what I did. When I got to the gym and saw that I couldn't take the class I wanted, I hopped on the treadmill and ran six miles. It was hard and I was tired. But I pushed through, and afterward, I felt as though nothing could stop me. I was powerful because I had fought all the obstacles like a warrior and won.

What about you? Are you going to let obstacles stand in your way? Are you going to let distractions stop you from being strong and healthy? Don't let anything get in the way of reaching your goals. Take those temptations and roadblocks as opportunities to be a champion. I know you can do it.

Something to Talk About

1. Have you had a bad day recently? How did it affect you?

2. Who has ultimate control over your mind?

3. Name some times when you have been tempted to quit but you didn't. How did it feel to push through?

Tip of the Day

Try talking to yourself to get motivated to do something you don't want to do. When you tell yourself what you're going to do, it reinforces that thought in your mind and makes it easier for you to do it.

DAY 69—FOCUS ON GOOD THINGS

—————————— A Note from Phil ——————————

Something to Think About

We've all had those days where it seems as if everything that can possibly go wrong does. We can't see anything good because we're focused on the bad things happening to us.

I want to remind us today to focus on the blessings—the good things—in our lives. We need to do this because our mind is like a magnifying glass. What happens when you look through one of those? The thing you're looking at gets bigger, right? Well, when we focus on the bad things in our lives, those things get bigger. And when we focus on the good things, those things will get bigger in our mind.

Here's how you can focus your mind on the positive. Remind yourself of your victories. If you hit a home run during a baseball game, got a good grade on a big test, or painted a picture that won a prize at the school art show, think about those things. Don't focus on the times you failed. Focus on the times you won.

Many people make goals and feel terrible when they don't reach them. But if you never set a goal, you wouldn't make any progress at all. If you set a goal and fall a little short, at least you got farther than you would have had you done nothing.

Life is good, and it is too short to focus on failures. Everyone has accomplished something they can celebrate. Celebrate those accomplishments today. And remember, you are a winner.

Something to Talk About

1. What are some victories in your life that you can celebrate?

2. Why should you focus on the good things in your life?

3. What are some things you can do when you're having a bad day that will help you feel better?

Tip of the Day

Write down something you would like to accomplish in your life. It could be to make the honor roll or to run a 5K race. Make some mini goals that can help you reach your big goal.

DAY 70—I AM AN ATHLETE

—————————— A Note from Phil ——————————

Something to Think About

When Amy and I started our own "Challenge," you could count on both hands how many times we had been in a gym in our entire lives. My athletic background was pretty minimal compared to the average man my age. Plus, I was carrying an extra 150 pounds on my frame. For sure, I could not be classified as athletic.

While we were at the ranch, our trainers always referred to us as athletes. Every time I heard that comparison, I laughed. I thought to myself, *They don't know anything about me. I am* not *an athlete.* If I ever said something like that out loud, our doctors and trainers would stop me right where I was and say, "Oh yes, you are." They explained that we were actually training as hard as the athletes who competed in the Olympics. That blew me away. We were also reminded that the extra weight we were all lugging around made our workouts even more challenging. Wow!

Through that experience, I realized that my life was no different from someone playing a professional sport or running a race. It was a competition. And I started believing that, yes, I was an athlete. I started viewing myself differently. I felt strong and motivated.

Take a look at yourself. What do you see? Do you believe there's an athlete hidden inside of you? I can tell you there is. Now own that truth and let the competition begin.

Something to Talk About

1. How do you see yourself in this "Challenge" to be healthy?

2. How can you have a better mind-set about who you really are?

3. How have you viewed yourself in the past? How will you view yourself in the future?

Tip of the Day

Pick one of your favorite athletes. Do some research to see what obstacles he or she had to overcome to be successful. This will encourage you to keep going.

Best Practices

Congratulations! You are almost at the end of the "Your Daily Fitness Challenge." We are so proud that you have stuck it out, and we're confident you have seen some amazing results. Here we will learn some key tips to maintaining good health throughout your entire life. These are best practices you will be able to use no matter how old you are or where you live.

—————————————— A Word from Amy ——————————————

Something to Think About

Recently I took our family to the beach for the week. We always look forward to going there to soak in some sun and relax. We leave the house just before daylight, and all the kids get their pillows and blankets and snuggle up together in the back of the van for the long drive down to the coast.

Imagine if I got in my car and started driving northwest when the beach is southeast. Do you think I would get to the beach if I kept going in the wrong direction? What if I hoped and prayed really hard that I would get there? Would that make a difference? Of course it wouldn't. There's a certain route I need to take to get where I want to go.

It's the same way with anything in life. Things don't just happen; you must do specific things to make them happen. If you want to make good grades, you have to study hard to get those A's. If you want to be healthy, you have to eat the right foods and be active.

When I was overweight and unhealthy, I had only myself to blame. I had traveled in the wrong direction with my diet and exercise habits for a very long time. But all I had to do was make a decision to "turn my car around" and change my bad habits into healthy ones. You can do the same thing. It's never too late to change direction and follow the road map to a healthier life.

Something to Talk About

1. What roads are you traveling down that may require you to turn around?

2. How can you support each other to make the needed changes discussed in the previous question?

3. What are some long-term consequences to your health for taking the wrong road?

Tip of the Day

You are on a road trip and have to go to the drive-thru to grab a bite to eat. Rather than guess at finding the healthiest item on the menu, look it up first. Many mobile phones have apps that list nutrition information for many fast-food restaurants.

DAY 72—HIT THE BOOST BUTTON

—————————————— A Word from Amy ——————————————

Something to Think About

How many of you like to play video games? I bet most of you do. My youngest son, Rhett, loves to play car racing games. One of his favorite features about these games is the "boost" button. He can push this button and make his car go super-crazy fast. When he pushes it, he laughs as he flies past the other cars.

The "boost" button on his game does to those cars what water does for our bodies. Did you know that when you drink water, it boosts your metabolism and gives you more energy? Water may seem boring compared to all the tasty juices, sodas, and other drinks out there, but it is the most powerful of all drinks. God created it to perfectly fit what our body needs.

Water hydrates us right down to our cells. It also boosts our liver's ability to change stored fat into energy that our body can use. It keeps us healthy and makes us feel good. It prevents us from being so hungry and satisfies cravings. Water is a super fuel for our bodies. Sodas and other sugary drinks actually make us thirsty, and the sugar, caffeine, and other chemicals in those drinks are bad for us. If you want to be healthier, make the choice to trade all the soda you drink for water. Go ahead, press the boost button.

Something to Talk About

1. What are some drinks that you may be drinking regularly that you can replace with water?

2. Why is water a "booster"?

3. Read the label on a soda can. What are some of the ingredients that might not be good for you? Discuss them.

Tip of the Day

Squeeze fresh lemon juice into your water. It will enhance the flavor and may be an aid in digestion.

DAY 73—GETTING YOUR ZZZZS

—————————— A Word from Amy ——————————

Something to Think About

Have you ever fought with your parents because you didn't want to take a nap or go to sleep when it was your bedtime? My mama told me that when I was a little girl, I didn't want to miss a thing, so I never wanted to sleep. Maybe you are like me and would rather go and go until you drop from exhaustion. But not getting enough sleep is not good for your health.

You need to get the right amount of sleep for a few reasons. Sleep helps our body and brain develop properly. Your brain needs sleep so that you can pay attention in school and remember what you're learning. Have you ever been in class and had a hard time focusing on what the teacher was saying? Well, you probably didn't get enough sleep the night before. Sleep also helps you to solve problems and be creative.

Our body needs sleep so we can grow big and strong. You may have heard that Popeye ate spinach to be strong, but I bet he also got a lot of sleep. Your muscles, skin, and even your bones need rest to be healthy.

One more thing. If you don't get enough sleep, your body can't fight off sickness very well. And I'm sure you hate being sick.

Toddlers need 10 to 12 hours of sleep a day, but when we get older we still need 8 hours a day to have the proper amount of rest. So the next time your parents tell you it's time for bed, snuggle up and get some shut-eye. Your body will thank you for it.

Something to Talk About

1. What are some reasons your brain needs sleep?

2. Why do you need sleep?

3. How many hours of sleep do you get per night? Should you be sleeping more?

Tip of the Day

Make sure your room is completely dark when you go to sleep. Light signals the brain that it's time to wake up, so cut off those lights.

DAY 74—PACKING A HEALTHY LUNCH

—————————— A Word from Amy ——————————

Something to Think About

I have three boys, and whenever we go to the grocery store, they beg me to buy junk food to put in their lunch bags for school. I always tell them no and that it is my job to make sure they stay healthy. If I let them eat chips, cookies, and other sugary treats for lunch, I wouldn't be doing my job. Here are some healthy things I usually pack in their lunch boxes.

- A piece of fruit—apples, oranges, bananas, grapes, or any kind they enjoy eating.

- Turkey, chicken, roast beef, or peanut butter sandwiches, making sure to include a source of protein and to use whole-wheat bread. I also use mustard rather than mayo because it is low in calories and has no unhealthy fat in it.

- String cheese or Greek yogurt. These snacks are a source of protein, calcium, and healthy fat.

- Almonds or some other kind of nuts. Nuts are a great source of healthy fat.

- Cut-up veggies. My kids especially love baby carrots. You can cut up broccoli, peppers, or cauliflower.

- Water. No lunch should be complete without it.

This is a sample of some healthy lunch-box ideas. Kick to the curb the snacks that are high in sugar and empty calories, and make sure your kids' lunch has the fuel they need to be strong, fit, and healthy.

Something to Talk About

1. What are some things in the list above that you would like to see in your lunch box?

2. What are some unhealthy things you are eating for lunch that you shouldn't be eating?

3. How can you make your lunches healthier?

Tip of the Day

Fill your water bottle mostly with ice in the morning before you pack it in your lunch box. By lunchtime, you'll have ice-cold water.

DAY 75—SHOPPING SMART

———————— A Word from Amy ————————

Something to Think About

Do you wish that money grew on trees? I know I do. It would be nice if we didn't have to think about how much something costs when we go shopping. Unfortunately, your parents have to work hard to make the money they use to buy things for you. That's why they need to shop smart to feed you healthy foods.

Parents, I highly recommend that you buy in bulk things you eat weekly. Items such as frozen chicken breasts, apples, brown rice, salsa, spinach, spices, fish, peanut butter, and oatmeal can be purchased at wholesale clubs for less money than buying them at the grocery store. Kids, help your parents clip coupons out of the newspaper so they can save money on items at the grocery store. And if you are shopping together, keep your eye on the sale signs and let your parents know what's on sale.

Don't beg your mom or dad to take you through the drive-thru or out to eat at a restaurant. Eating out just one time a week can cost the same amount as a week's worth of groceries. Also, you don't always know what you're eating (or how healthy your meal is) at a restaurant because you aren't in control of the ingredients. Wouldn't you rather cook a meal together and enjoy it around your table as a family? If you do, you'll have more money to spend on other things, such as going to the movies or even taking a vacation.

And don't impulse shop. Go to the grocery store and buy only what you need. You'll stop yourself from spending more money than you need to.

Something to Talk About

1. What are some ways you can help your parents save money on their groceries?

2. Why is eating out a lot not good for your budget?

3. Why is impulse shopping bad?

Tip of the Day

Many websites, such as www.couponmom.com, teach how to save extra money using coupons. Find other sites and use them as a resource to help you eat healthier for less money.

DAY 76—TOP 10 THINGS TO DO NOW

—————————— A Word from Amy ——————————

Something to Think About

Why do your teachers at school give you tests? To make sure you're learning what he or she is teaching you, right? Unless it's a pop quiz, you always have a chance to review your notes. You've learned a lot of tips reading this book. Today's "Challenge" is a review of some of those tips plus a few new ones. Make sure you study so you can pass your test to being healthy.

1. Drink a glass of water as soon as you wake up in the morning. It will start your body moving and flush out your pancreas.

2. Drink water all day. It will give you energy and keep you hydrated.

3. Kick the salt. It's amazing how good food tastes once you get rid of all the salt in your food. Use salt substitute if you need to.

4. Start eating fruits and vegetables (enough said!). Over 95 percent of Americans do not get enough fruits and vegetables. Don't be a part of that statistic.

5. Try to eat four to six small meals and snacks each day. Don't starve yourself. Fuel your body.

6. Combine protein, carbohydrates, and a small dose of natural fat in each meal.

7. Eat like a king for breakfast. This should be your largest meal of the day.

8. Activate your body. Get at least 30 minutes of movement in every day. Ride your bike, walk, or play sports. It doesn't matter what you do as long as you keep moving.

9. Cut out the soda. Even diet soda is bad for you because it's made with artificial sweeteners that aren't good for you.

10. Believe in yourself! You can do it. The power to change is within you.

Something to Talk About

1. Why is diet soda as bad for you as regular soda?

2. What should you combine with every meal and snack?

3. At what point during your day should you start drinking water?

Tip of the Day

Learning is a wonderful thing. On your path to good health, check out health-and-fitness books and magazines and keep learning more on how you can be healthy.

DAY 77—IDEAS FOR TRAVELING

———————— A Word from Amy ————————

Something to Think About

Do you like going on vacation? Of course you do. Everyone does! It's fun to get away with your family and have a good time. I encourage you, however, not to forget about being healthy even when you're away from home. We never need a vacation from eating better and exercising more. Even when we're far from home, we can always take time to be active and make sure we're eating good foods.

Vacation should be a relaxing time, but you should make sure to include activity while you're away. If you're staying at the beach or in the mountains, there are plenty of fun things to do to keep active. You can run on the beach, swim, bike, hike, ski, or surf. These are just a few activities that can make vacation memorable. After all, what's the point of going somewhere if you're going to sit around a hotel room and play video games all day. You could do that at home.

Also, just because you're away from home doesn't mean you can eat lots of junk food. It's okay to have an occasional treat, but too much is not good. My kids like to go out for ice cream when we go on vacation, but we don't do it every day. It's a special treat reserved for one night.

Parents, be sure to pack healthy snacks for your family just as you do when you're at home. And when you go out to eat, make healthy choices. Vacation is no time to make an excuse to have unhealthy habits. Stay on track and have fun.

Something to Talk About

1. What are some active things you can do on vacation that are healthy?

2. What are some ways to avoid eating junk food and playing video games when you're away?

3. How can you eat healthy on vacation?

Tip of the Day

Before you go away, take some time to plan fun activities with your family. Do some research and see what neat things are offered in the area you are traveling.

DAY 78—DON'T GET DEFEETED

—————————— A Word from Amy ——————————

Something to Think About

If you were an astronaut, you wouldn't go to the moon without a space suit. If you were a soldier, you wouldn't go to war without your weapons. And if you were an athlete, you wouldn't exercise without the right shoes. Well, you *are* an athlete, so you need to take care of your feet.

Taking care of your feet means wearing the right shoes. When you're playing sports, walking, or riding your bike, flip-flops just won't cut it. They're way too flimsy. You need to wear the right athletic shoes. Ask your mom or dad to take you to a store that specializes in running shoes. The people who work there can look at your feet and properly fit you with the right shoe. They can tell you if you have a foot with a high arch or if you have a flat foot. Different shoes work with different feet.

You may find that if you haven't been very active and you start doing more activity than usual, you may feel some pain in your feet and knees. If this happens, you need to remember RICE: Rest, Ice, Compress, and Elevate. Rest your feet, put ice packs on them, wrap them up, and elevate them (or put them up). If you do this at the first sign of pain, it will help you protect your legs and feet from injury.

Something to Talk About

1. What does RICE stand for?

2. Why should you have the right shoes when you are exercising?

3. What can a store that specializes in running shoes do that other stores might not be able to do?

Tip of the Day

When you're doing RICE, you can use a bag of frozen vegetables, such as peas or corn, instead of an ice pack. The cold vegetables wrap around your leg better, and you can eat them later.

DAY 79—EAT BETWEEN MEALS

—————————— A Word from Amy ——————————

Something to Think About

Has your mother ever told you not to eat between meals? Well, I'm not telling you not to listen to your parents, but did you know that the right snacks are an important part of staying healthy? Eating between meals is good for you provided you're eating the right foods. We talked earlier about how your body is like a car that needs gas to run. Well, healthy snacks are the gas that keeps you going.

When I talk about snacks, I'm not talking about cookies, candy, or chips. I'm talking about nutritious foods, such as fruits, veggies, and nuts, that are good fuel for your body. Keep in mind that you should always mix proteins, carbohydrates, and fats. Here are some examples of snacks we eat regularly:

- apple and almonds
- Wasa cracker and Laughing Cow cheese
- yogurt with fruit
- orange slices and pistachios
- carrots, broccoli, celery, and hummus

- blue corn chips and salsa
- granola or Kashi with almond milk
- air-popped popcorn with nuts and fruit
- rice cake with peanut butter
- banana and almond butter

Eating snacks such as these twice a day will keep your energy level stable. Pack some in your lunch box so you can have a snack in the afternoon. If you play with friends or go to sports practice, make sure you take a healthy snack with you.

Don't skip any meals on this challenge. Eat, but eat well.

Something to Talk About

1. What are some snacks you like from the list above? Can you name some of your favorites that aren't on the list?

2. Why do you need to eat between meals?

3. What three things should you mix with each snack?

Tip of the Day

Pack several snacks in individual bags ahead of time so that if you're in a hurry, you can grab them and go.

DAY 80—EATING OUT

———— A Word from Amy ————

Something to Think About

Do you love to go out to eat with your family? I know my family does. When you're trying to get healthier and eat things that are good for you, going to a restaurant can seem like a challenge. What do you order? What is healthy? Can you just have a slice of pizza? Here are some tips that might help you and your family make better choices when you go to a restaurant:

- Make friends with your server. Let them know you're trying to eat healthier, and they may recommend some healthy menu items. Ask if they have a nutrition guide.

- Don't eat the bread that usually comes before a meal. Tell the waiter to take away the bread basket as soon as you sit down.

- Drink water instead of soda. Water is also free, so you can save money while being healthy!

- If you have to choose a side item, choose rice or steamed veggies over french fries or mashed potatoes.

- Order your meats or fish grilled instead of fried.

- Avoid creamy sauces, gravy, and oils that add fat.

- Skip the dessert.

- Eat sensibly. When you get your food, immediately pack up half of it to take home. This way you can clean your plate without eating too much.

It's easy to overeat when eating out in restaurants, so be careful. Order healthy meals in a healthy amount wherever you go.

Something to Talk About

1. What should you do when you get your food?

2. What extras should you avoid on your food?

3. Name some examples of healthy options for side items.

Tip of the Day

Before you go out to eat, go online and see if you can find a copy of the restaurant's menu or nutrition guide. Spend a few minutes deciding what might be a healthy option to order.

Make a Difference

One of the greatest things we can do in this life is to give back to others. We can do this in many different ways. We can help someone in need by giving them money, volunteering our time, or even encouraging them. Be inspired to make a difference in the lives of others, and be a blessing.

DAY 81—YOU ARE A SEED

--------------------------------- A Word from Amy ---------------------------------

Something to Think About

Everyone wants their life to count. God placed inside each of us the desire to do great things. I like to think about my life as a little seed planted in the world. God has a purpose for my life, and as I grow and try my best to be led by Him, I will do what I am made to do. One purpose we all share is to help other people. We are all created to make a difference in the lives of others.

One way we can make a difference is by sharing our gifts. No, I'm not talking about a beautifully wrapped package. Do you know we all have something special we can do that someone else may have trouble doing? You might be good in math and your brother might be good in English. You can help your brother in math because it's easy for you. Maybe you're a really good artist. You could draw a picture for someone to cheer them up. There is always something we can do to help someone else.

The Bible says in Galatians 6:7-10 that we reap what we sow. This is a spiritual law drawn from a natural law that says when we plant something, the plant that grows from it is determined by the kind of seed we planted. What we put into the ground, we will get back. If we plant a watermelon seed, we will get a watermelon.

Think about what you are sowing into the lives of other people. Are you sowing seeds of kindness? Are you sowing seeds of love? Are you sowing seeds of a good attitude? Whatever you plant will be what you will harvest. So be sure to plant good things.

Something to Talk About

1. Why is it good to do things for other people?

2. What does making a difference in the lives of others have to do with being fit?

3. What are your gifts that you can use to help others?

Tip of the Day

Take a minute to think about the gifts you have that you could use to help others. Look for an opportunity to use one of those gifts to help someone today.

DAY 82—GIVING

A Word from Amy

Something to Think About

One part of this journey into good health is to use what you've learned to make a difference in the lives of others. I am truly blessed to have a wonderful sister-in-law who is a giver. Recently, she gave of her time to help me move and even organized all my kitchen cabinets. She is always there if we need someone to watch the kids. But the cherry on top of her giving sundae was when she gave me almost an entire wardrobe when she sorted out her closet. She has great taste in clothes, and some of the items she gave me were ones I always liked when she wore them.

Have you ever had a friend who gave you something really special? Did you feel warm and fuzzy inside? Did it make you feel valuable? Wouldn't it be nice if you could make others feel that way? Well, you can.

You have the power to make others feel special by being a giver. Just think of some things you can give to others. Do you have a special talent you can share? Can you say an encouraging word to make someone's day? Can you spend time with someone who is sad?

When you're a role model to your friends and family, you are making a difference. See, it's easy to do! Keep up the good work and keep making a difference.

Something to Talk About

1. Has someone given or done something to you that made you feel special?

2. What is something you can give to others to make them feel special?

3. How can you use this fitness challenge to help others?

Tip of the Day

Clean out your closet. Give away some of your old things to people who might need them. One man's trash is another man's treasure.

DAY 83—SERVING OTHERS

———————————— A Word from Amy ————————————

Something to Think About

Like many students, when I was in college and Bible school I worked as a waitress. It was a tough job. I spent long hours on my feet, carried heavy trays, and relied on the kindness of strangers to give me good tips, since that was where most of my earnings came from. Many of the waitresses would grumble and complain about the customers when they were out of earshot. I'll admit, it was tempting to do if someone was rude or they didn't leave you a tip.

One day at work I started to feel bad about talking about the customers. I decided to change my attitude and serve them as Christ would want me to. It was amazing that with this mental change, I started enjoying my job so much more. It also made a difference in the tips I got. I started making more money than any of the other girls in the restaurant.

When we do things God's way, we are rewarded for it. He made us, and He knows what is best for us. We are made to serve and to help each other. So find ways today to help make the lives of the people you come in contact with better. There are plenty of negative complainers in the world. Be the positive light that makes a difference in a good way.

Something to Talk About

1. What are some ways you can serve others in your life?

2. What tasks can you do with a better attitude?

3. What happens when you grumble and complain?

Tip of the Day

When you go to a restaurant and you get good service, make sure you give the waitress a generous tip. Remember that many of them are taking care of their families with the money you leave on the table.

DAY 84—SERVING YOUR COMMUNITY

A Word from Amy

Something to Think About

What does it mean to be a good citizen? Does it mean that you need to say the Pledge of Allegiance every day and put your hand over your heart when you hear the national anthem? That may be part of it, but being a good citizen is about serving the people in your community who need your help.

Serving others is another way you can make a difference. Here are a few ideas how you can do that. You could pick up trash on the side of the road or plant trees. You could volunteer at a nursing home and read to an older person. You could serve at a soup kitchen or you could give clothes and food to a relief organization. There are a number of ways to give back to your community.

When my son Rhett was younger, he was a part of an organization called the Miracle League. This organization was for kids with special needs who couldn't play regular baseball. They had a special field made of recycled tires so that wheelchairs could roll on it. Each child had a buddy who helped them hit the ball and assisted them around the bases. My older sons decided to become buddies for the team. They enjoyed helping the kids, and it helped them to be thankful for their health.

Think about how you can help those around you in your neighborhood or school. Enlist the help of your teachers or parents to give you some ideas. You'll be blessed when you use your time to make a difference.

Something to Talk About

1. What does it mean to be a good citizen?

2. Is there an organization you would like to serve?

3. In what ways do you think helping your community can also help you?

Tip of the Day

Picking up trash around your neighborhood is a good way to start helping your community. Grab a couple of your friends and do it today.

DAY 85—THANKFULNESS

———————— A Word from Amy ————————

Something to Think About

The Bible is filled with verses that tell us to be thankful. Several passages talk about prayer and thanksgiving in the same sentence. Thanking God for things He has done or has given us shows Him how grateful we are. It's funny, but the more thankful we become, the more things we find to be thankful for.

I'll be honest. Some things in my life I am not thankful for. I am not thankful for bills that come every month. I am not thankful for dishwashers that don't work. I am not thankful for fingerprints on glass or for family members who don't always get along. However, I am thankful for the house I live in that creates the bills. I am thankful that I have food that makes our dishes dirty. I am thankful for my kids, the ones who make the dirty fingerprints. And I am thankful for the family that I love.

Focus on being grateful for big things and little things, such as food and shelter, nice teachers at school, a loving family, good friends, and even the toys you have. Nothing is too little to appreciate.

What do you have to be thankful for? Start thinking about that question. Having a thankful attitude also makes your light shine brighter to those around you and helps them have a better day.

Something to Talk About

1. Name three things you are thankful for.

2. How does being thankful make your day better?

3. Do you thank God every day? How about your parents?

Tip of the Day

Singing praise and worship songs is a great way to thank God for what He has done for us. We can always be grateful to Him for saving us and giving us the gift of His only Son.

DAY 86—WHAT WE LEAVE BEHIND

A Word from Amy

Something to Think About

My dad has a creepy obsession with touring graveyards and reading tombstones. He has convinced me a few times to go with him on these adventures. Although I'm not as excited about this hobby as he is, I am interested in reading the tombstones. It's amazing that a life is minimized to the dates of birth and death and maybe a few words, such as "loving mother" or "caring brother," on a piece of stone. Every time I have visited these places with my dad, it made me think about what I want people to remember about me when I die.

What do you want people to remember about you? What do you want to leave behind? You will make a mark on this world if you made a difference in the lives of others. Whether good or bad, people are remembered by how their lives influenced those around them.

I want my life to be one that has helped people be better. I want to have helped my kids to be the best they can be. I want my friends to be able to say I was there for them when they needed me. I want my husband to know I loved him with all my heart. I want to help others have the best life they can have by sharing with them the blessings I've been given. I want you to be inspired to know that you can be the best you can be.

Make it your mission to help others, and you will leave a rich legacy.

Something to Talk About

1. What would you like your tombstone to say about you?

2. What can you do to make an impact on your family or friends?

3. What kind of legacy are you leaving right now?

Tip of the Day

Sit down with a grandparent and ask them to tell you about their life. You might learn something about them that surprises you.

DAY 87—BE AN INSPIRATION

———————— A Word from Amy ————————

Something to Think About

Have you ever had someone tell you that you inspired them to do something? Do you know what that means? To inspire someone means to breathe hope into them. It's a wonderful gift to be able to give someone hope. If you have a friend who is discouraged and you say something to make them feel better, you are inspiring them.

You can also be an inspiration by setting a good example. When you do the right things and are kind and helpful, people take notice. You can inspire other people just by being the best you can be. Giving to others, thinking of others before yourself, and simply living out the Golden Rule are great ways to be an inspiration. When you do these things, your friends can see Christ through your actions.

When it comes to your health, people are watching you too. People notice when you eat right and are active. You can inspire your friends to make the right choices just by leading a healthy lifestyle. When you go to school and eat an apple instead of chips or drink water instead of soda, your friends will notice. My kids have watched how I have changed my eating habits and started exercising more, and they have decided to do the same thing. And this happened not because of what I said to them, but because I was modeling the right actions.

Do you want to inspire other people? Then do the right things, and others will surely follow your lead.

Something to Talk About

1. What does it mean to be an inspiration?

2. How can you set a good example for your friends?

3. What things can you do to inspire people to be healthier?

Tip of the Day

Call a friend today and encourage them.

DAY 88—SOMETIMES YOU GET MORE THAN YOU GIVE

—————————— A Word from Amy ——————————

Something to Think About

I was involved in a community organization that gave food and gift baskets to needy families over the holidays. I had lived a fairly comfortable life growing up. I didn't have the latest fashions or the newest toys, but I wasn't poor by any means. My perspective of poverty completely changed when we were delivering the gift baskets to these families.

I walked through the front door of one family's home and was shocked at how worn out their home was. There were even holes in the floor so large you could see the dirt underneath the house. In the corner, I saw three children huddled around a black-and-white television that barely got reception. They were covered with dirt and grime and looked so sad. The father was in bed, too sick to get up. The mother told us that because her husband was ill, he was out of work; she had to stay home with the children, so they had no income. It broke my heart.

I'll never forget how excited this woman and her kids were to see our gifts. It made my heart so happy that even though I couldn't change their situation, I could do a little something to bring joy to their day. Suddenly, the problems I had seemed very small. I saw my life in a completely different light and had a better attitude about appreciating all I had.

Being able to give to that family was the best gift I got for Christmas that year. When you make a difference in others, you get a lot more than what you give.

Something to Talk About

1. Have you ever done something for someone and got more in return?

2. What did you learn from the story about this family in need?

3. Why do you think God is pleased when we give?

Tip of the Day

To avoid blisters when you do a lot of walking or running, wear socks with sections for your toes. It will keep your tootsies from rubbing together and will enable you to run more comfortably.

DAY 89—THE MULTIPLICATION FACTOR

A Word from Amy

Something to Think About

Have you ever heard the phrase, "You can't out give God"? I can tell you with certainty that this statement is true because I've experienced it. When we were living in Washington State, a guest minister visited our church and talked about the importance of giving. I was so excited to give, until I realized I didn't have any money. I knew there must be something I could give to God. Immediately I thought about a beautiful diamond ring my mother-in-law had given to me. I knew that was what I had to donate in the next offering. I did it without telling anybody.

What happened next may sound crazy to some of you, but I swear it's true. Within the next week, someone had given me a car, a computer, and another diamond ring. Three separate people told me they felt led to give these things to me. I was so excited that I gave the car and the ring away to other people I thought needed them more than I did. Within two weeks, someone else gave me a newer car, and I got some money in the mail. It was unbelievable. I was so excited to keep giving—to help others and to thank God—and I learned I couldn't out give God. He is the ultimate gift giver.

I know we don't give for the purpose of receiving, but this happens to be a law in the Bible. Jesus tells us, "Give, and it will be given to you" (Luke 6:38). Remember, you can't out give God. Give your time, talents, and gifts to someone today, and test out this law for yourself.

Something to Talk About

1. Have you ever known you were supposed to give someone something when it was really hard?
2. Have you ever given something and seen God's blessings come back to you?
3. What does the saying, "You can't out give God" mean to you?

Tip of the Day

Planting a garden is a living example of the law of sowing and reaping. When you plant one tomato plant, you may get a hundred tomatoes. Try this in your backyard.

DAY 90—RECEIVING BLESSING

A Word from Amy

Something to Think About

We have talked so much about giving to others, but what do we do when others give to us? I used to feel bad when someone would give me something if I didn't have something to give in return. I would feel guilty until I had evened the score. One day someone wanted to give me something, and I refused to accept it. But my friend said something that made me change my mind: "Why are you going to rob me of a blessing?"

I had never thought about it that way. When we don't allow someone to give to us, we are keeping them from being blessed. We are keeping them from sowing their seed that will cause them to grow a crop. We know that we need to be good givers, but we need to be good receivers too.

The same thing applies when someone pays us a compliment. It took me the longest time to just say "thank you" when someone told me I did a good job or I looked nice. I would try to deflect the compliment by saying, "Oh, it was nothing," or "Oh, this old thing?" When people pay us compliments, they're trying to do something nice for us. We need to receive that blessing.

Accepting blessings is another great way to make a difference in other people's lives. God gave us the best gift ever when He gave Jesus to save the world from sin. We need to accept that gift above all.

Be thankful for good things that come your way and be a good receiver.

Something to Talk About

1. What is the best gift ever given?

2. Why do we need to be good receivers?

3. What does it mean to "rob someone of a blessing"?

Tip of the Day

Practice saying "thank you" when someone pays you a compliment. It's a good way to learn to be a receiver.

Conclusion

Congratulations! Not only did you complete *The Amazing Fitness Adventure for Your Kids*, you have also embarked on a whole new chapter in your life. I'm sure you and your family feel better, healthier, and have more energy than when you started this challenge.

We are so proud that you realize how important good health is to you and your kids and that you have taken the appropriate steps to make this a priority in your family. We encourage you to take what you have learned in this book and continue to walk the journey of good health. Just because these 90 days are up doesn't mean you can go back to your old lifestyle habits. Keep moving forward. Keep taking the right steps and making the right decisions when it comes to nutrition and fitness.

Make a difference and leave a legacy for others to follow in your footsteps. We know you can do it!

Appendix A

Shopping List

FRUITS and VEGETABLES

- ☐ Blueberries
- ☐ Strawberries
- ☐ Blackberries
- ☐ Raspberries
- ☐ Apples (all varieties)
- ☐ Lemon
- ☐ Lime
- ☐ Bananas
- ☐ Grapefruit
- ☐ Artichokes
- ☐ Spaghetti squash (not banana squash)
- ☐ Carrots
- ☐ Brussels sprouts
- ☐ Asparagus
- ☐ Broccoli
- ☐ Cauliflower
- ☐ Bell pepper (orange, red, green, yellow)
- ☐ Celery

- ☐ Cucumber
- ☐ Daikon
- ☐ Cilantro
- ☐ Mint
- ☐ Ginger root
- ☐ Endive
- ☐ Eggplant
- ☐ Garlic
- ☐ Jicama
- ☐ Lettuce (all varieties)
- ☐ Spinach (regular or baby)
- ☐ Onions
- ☐ Dried seaweed
- ☐ Sprouts
- ☐ Zucchini
- ☐ Tomato
- ☐ Cherry tomato
- ☐ Mushrooms
- ☐ Stir-fry vegetables (frozen)
- ☐ Green beans

RICE/BREADS/CARBS

- ☐ Wild long-grain rice
- ☐ Brown short-grain rice
- ☐ Whole-grain quinoa
- ☐ Brown-rice pasta
- ☐ Ezekiel low-sodium bread

- ☐ Ezekiel buns
- ☐ Ezekiel tortillas
- ☐ Corn tortilla
- ☐ Low-carb whole-wheat tortillas
- ☐ 100 percent whole-wheat bread

☐ Steel-cut oatmeal
☐ Quaker low-sugar oatmeal
☐ Quaker weight-control oatmeal
☐ Weetabix

☐ Kashi GOLEAN waffles
☐ Kashi GOLEAN cereal
☐ All-Bran low-sodium cereal

BEANS

☐ Chickpeas
☐ Edamame blanched-shelled soybeans (frozen)
☐ Fat-free low-sodium black beans
☐ Dried lentils

☐ Great northern beans
☐ Red beans
☐ Black beans
☐ Low-sodium hummus

NUTS

☐ Dry-roasted almonds
☐ Raw walnuts
☐ Raw pecans
☐ Raw cashews

☐ Organic or all-natural peanut butter
☐ Hemp seed nuts
☐ Flax seeds or fiber

MEATS/FISH/PROTEINS

☐ Wild Alaskan salmon (not farm raised)
☐ Tilapia
☐ Tuna steaks (albacore and ahi)
☐ Tuna (canned, no salt)
☐ Alaskan black cod
☐ Catfish
☐ Alaskan halibut
☐ Chicken breast (organic, boneless, skinless, raw)
☐ Turkey (organic, ground turkey

breast and raw [previously frozen OK])
☐ Ground turkey
☐ Chicken (ground white meat)
☐ No-salt sliced turkey breast
☐ Turkey burgers
☐ Turkey sausage
☐ Uncured, no-nitrite turkey bacon
☐ Low-sodium roast beef
☐ Grass-fed beef (all kinds)

DAIRY

☐ AllWhites 100% Liquid Egg Whites
☐ Omega-3 whole eggs
☐ Nonfat sour cream
☐ Organic fat-free milk
☐ FAGE Total 2% Greek yogurt
☐ Organic fat-free yogurt (FAGE Total 0%)

☐ Reduced-fat string cheese
☐ Laughing Cow Light Cheese Wedges
☐ Cottage cheese (low fat)
☐ Tzatziki Greek-strained yogurt dip

CONDIMENTS/DRESSINGS/OILS/SAUCES

- ☐ While balsamic vinegar
- ☐ Balsamic vinegar
- ☐ Rice wine vinegar
- ☐ No-sugar, low-sodium organic pasta sauce
- ☐ No-carb BBQ sauce and ketchup
- ☐ Galileo low-fat salad dressings (all flavors)
- ☐ Mustard (all varieties)
- ☐ Mayo (fat-free)
- ☐ Low-sodium, organic chicken broth
- ☐ Extra virgin olive oil
- ☐ Flaxseed oil
- ☐ I Can't Believe It's Not Butter Spray
- ☐ Cooking sprays
- ☐ Salsa

SEASONINGS and SPICES

- ☐ Allspice
- ☐ Basil
- ☐ Oregano
- ☐ Curry
- ☐ Turmeric
- ☐ Chili powder
- ☐ Crushed red pepper
- ☐ Dill
- ☐ Cinnamon
- ☐ Rosemary
- ☐ Pepper
- ☐ Cavender's Salt Free Greek Seasoning
- ☐ Old Bay Seasoning
- ☐ Morton Salt Substitute
- ☐ Chef Paul Prudhomme's Magic Salt-Free Seasoning
- ☐ Mrs. Dash Salt-Free Seasoning Blends

SWEETENERS

- ☐ Xylitol packets
- ☐ XyloSweet
- ☐ Stevia extract
- ☐ No-sugar, low glycemic jelly

COFFEE/TEAS

- ☐ Coffee (organic)
- ☐ Green tea (organic)
- ☐ Dandelion tea
- ☐ Lemon ginger tea (organic)
- ☐ Milk thistle tea (organic)
- ☐ Sparkling mineral water
- ☐ Honest Tea (black assam tea)

NONDAIRY and JUICES

- ☐ Organic rice milk, almond milk, or soy milk
- ☐ Unsweetened cranberry juice (such as Knudsen Just Cranberry)
- ☐ Labrada CarbWatchers Lean Body shakes (vanilla and chocolate)
- ☐ Emergen-C vitamin drink mixes

SNACKS

- ☐ Blue corn tortilla chips
- ☐ Snapea Crisps
- ☐ Wasa Whole Wheat Crispbread
- ☐ Streit's Matzos Unsalted
- ☐ Cuban crackers
- ☐ Sugar-free gelatin
- ☐ Whipped cream
- ☐ Sugar-free pudding

Top 10 List of Kids' Favorite Foods (Made Healthy)

1. Macaroni-and-Cheese Pie

Ingredients:
  32 ounces whole-wheat elbow macaroni
  3 egg whites
  3 cups skim milk
  3 cups shredded cheese (one-half skim mozzarella cheese and one-half Cabot's reduced-fat cheddar cheese, mixed together)
  Dash of salt

Directions:
1. Preheat oven to 350 degrees F (175 degrees C).

2. Bring a large pot of lightly salted water to a boil. Add macaroni and cook for 8 to 10 minutes or until tender; drain.

3. Beat egg whites and milk together. Pour half of the cooked macaroni into 9x13-inch baking dish. Cover macaroni with half of the cheese. Pour remaining macaroni into baking dish leaving a little room at the top. Cover with remaining cheese. Pour egg mixture over macaroni.

4. Bake in a preheated over for an hour or until a knife inserted comes out clean.

Makes 6 servings

2. Healthy Spaghetti

Ingredients:

    1 pound lean ground turkey
    1 28-ounce can diced tomatoes
    1 cup green pepper, finely chopped
    1 cup onion, finely chopped
    1 cup mushrooms, sliced
    1 tablespoon minced garlic
    1 teaspoon Italian seasoning
    ½ teaspoon black pepper
    1 pound whole-wheat spaghetti, uncooked
    Nonstick cooking spray

Directions:

1. Coat large skillet with nonstick spray. Preheat over high heat.

2. Add turkey and cook, stirring occasionally, for 5 minutes. Drain and discard fat.

3. Stir in tomatoes with juice, green pepper, mushrooms, onion, garlic, Italian seasoning, and black pepper. Bring to boil. Reduce heat and simmer covered for 15 minutes, stirring occasionally. Remove cover and simmer for added 15 minutes.

4. Cook spaghetti. Drain well.

5. Serve sauce over spaghetti.

Makes 6 servings

3. Tacos

Ingredients:

    1 pound ground chicken or turkey (you can substitute
        black beans for meat)
    Chili powder, salt, and pepper (to taste)
    1 package of taco shells
    Reduced-fat cheddar cheese
    Shredded lettuce or spinach
    1 tomato, diced
    1 onion, chopped

1 cup sliced black olives
1 cup FAGE Greek yogurt (in place of sour cream)
Salsa (recipe below)
Guacamole (recipe below)

Directions:
1. Brown the ground chicken or turkey in a frying pan over medium-high heat. Add chili powder, salt, and pepper to taste.

2. Fill each taco with meat. My family prefers to add the other ingredients buffet style because they can choose the condiments they like the most. I like to make a taco salad for myself (spinach, meat, cheese, tomatoes, black olives, salsa, black beans, and a few tortilla chips over the top for crunch.)

* You can also use shredded chicken in place of beef or black beans. Simply throw some chicken breasts, chili powder, salt, and pepper in a Crock-Pot or slow cooker on high for about 4 hours or low for 6 to 8 hours. Shred the chicken with a fork before serving as part of a taco meal.

Makes 10 to 12 tacos

Ingredients for homemade salsa:
1 large tomato, chopped
1 small onion, chopped
Cilantro to taste
2 jalapeños, chopped and the seeds removed
Salt and pepper

Directions:
We use a mini food processor that we got for about $15. You can make the salsa or guacamole and store it in the same container. And it's easy to clean. Put all the salsa ingredients in the food processor and mix until it reaches your desired consistency. You can serve with tacos or blue corn tortilla chips.

Ingredients for homemade guacamole
2 ripe avocados
½ cup red onion, minced
1-2 jalapeño peppers, seeds removed, minced
2 tablespoons cilantro, finely chopped
1 tablespoon of fresh lime or lemon juice
½ teaspoon coarse salt
Dash black pepper
½ ripe tomato, chopped

Directions:
Mix all ingredients in your mini food processor to the desired consistency. Serve with tacos or blue corn tortilla chips.

4. Hamburgers and Fries

Ingredients for burgers:
1 pound ground turkey or chicken
1 egg white
¼ cup chopped onion
½ cup spinach
¼ cup old-fashioned oatmeal

Directions:
1. Mix all ingredients together and form patties. Spray a pan with nonstick cooking spray and cook patties until done.
2. Serve with desired condiments. We suggest mustard rather than mayo and ketchup for a healthier condiment. Lettuce, tomato, onion, and pickles are all great condiments to add. We also serve our burgers on whole-wheat buns or the 100-calorie flat buns, as most of the sugar and empty calories are found in white bread.
3. Serve with french fries (below).

Makes 5 burgers

Ingredients for french fries:
   3 large sweet potatoes, peeled and sliced into fries
   Nonstick cooking spray
   Cayenne pepper
   Salt
   Spray butter
   Honey or sugar-free maple syrup (if desired)

Directions for french fries:
1. Preheat oven to 350 degrees.

2. Spray a baking sheet with nonstick cooking spray and put the sliced sweet potatoes on the sheet. Spray with spray butter and sprinkle with cayenne pepper and salt.

3. Cook for 15 minutes or until tender. Baking time will be determined by how thick or thin you slice your potatoes. To add a sweeter taste, drizzle a little honey or maple syrup over the top 2 minutes before you take them out of the oven. You can also substitute cinnamon for the cayenne pepper, if desired.

Makes 4 servings

5. Blueberry Protein Pancake Breakfast

Ingredients:
   2 cups whole-wheat instant pancake mix
   ½ cup water
   1 container blueberry Greek yogurt
   Flaxseed and wheat germ (optional)
   Turkey bacon

Directions:
1. Spray frying pan with nonstick cooking spray and cook turkey bacon. Set it to the side.

2. Spray a griddle or separate frying pan with nonstick cooking spray. Mix pancake mix and water and a container of

blueberry yogurt together. Sneak flaxseed and wheat germ into pancakes to make them even healthier.

3. Cook until golden brown. Serve with turkey bacon.

Makes 12 small pancakes

6. Golden Pancakes

Ingredients:

> 1 cup oatmeal, uncooked
> 6 egg whites
> 1 cup fat-free cottage cheese
> ¼ teaspoon vanilla
> ¼ teaspoon cinnamon
> 2 packets of xylitol or stevia

Directions:

1. Mix all ingredients together.
2. Cook batter on a griddle sprayed with nonstick cooking spray.
3. Top with ½ cup sugar-free maple syrup

Makes 12 silver-dollar pancakes; 4 servings (3 pancakes per serving)

7. Mashed "Potatoes"

Ingredients:

> 1 large head of cauliflower
> 1 cup skim milk
> 1 wedge of Laughing Cow cheese (original)
> Salt and pepper

Directions:

1. Cook cauliflower until fork tender.
2. Cut cauliflower into small pieces and mix with remaining ingredients until smooth.

* If you like garlic mashed potatoes, you can also mix in ¼ teaspoon of minced garlic.

Makes 6 ½-cup servings

8. Chicken Nuggets

Ingredients:
½ cup skim milk
1 teaspoon poultry seasoning
1 cup cornflakes, crushed
1½ tablespoons onion powder
1½ tablespoons garlic powder
2 teaspoons black pepper
2 teaspoons red pepper, crushed
5 skinless chicken breasts (cut into nuggets or strips)
Dash (or 2) paprika
Nonstick cooking spray

Directions:
1. Preheat oven to 350 degrees F.

2. Add ½ teaspoon poultry seasoning to milk.

3. Combine other ½ teaspoon poultry seasoning and all other spices with cornflake crumbs and place in plastic bag.

4. Wash chicken and pat dry. Dip chicken into milk, shake to remove excess, then quickly shake in bag with seasoning and crumbs.

5. Refrigerate for 1 hour.

6. Remove from refrigerator and sprinkle lightly with paprika for color.

7. Evenly space chicken on baking sheet sprayed with nonstick cooking spray.

8. Cover with aluminum foil and bake for 40 minutes. Remove foil and check to make sure it is cooked throughout. The size of your nuggets will determine the cooking time.

Makes 7 servings (about 4 nuggets per serving)

9. "Ice Cream" Sundae

Ingredients:
2 containers of FAGE yogurt

Xylitol or stevia sweetener

2 scoops PB2 powdered peanut butter (you can order this at www.bellplantation.com)

Strawberries, bananas, or raspberries, chopped (any fruit will do)

Almond slivers

Directions:

1. Mix yogurt with 2 packets of stevia or xylitol sweetener.

2. Add PB2 powdered peanut butter.

3. Freeze for 1 hour or until slightly firm.

4. Scoop in a container and top with fruit and nuts.

* If your children like vanilla ice cream, substitute vanilla flavoring for the PB2. You can also add whatever fruit your children like best.

Makes 4 servings

10. Individual Pizza

Ingredients:

6 English muffins

2 cups prepared pizza sauce

¼ cup green or red bell pepper, cubed

¼ cup onion

¼ cup sliced black olives

1/8 teaspoon dried Italian herb seasoning

1 cup part-skim mozzarella cheese

½ cup grated Parmesan cheese

Turkey bacon or sausage cooked and crumbled (optional)

Directions:

1. Preheat oven to 350 degrees.

2. Slice English muffins in half and place them on a baking sheet.

3. Spoon pizza sauce on top of muffins.

4. Add peppers and onions.

5. Sprinkle herb seasoning on top.

6. If desired, add turkey bacon or sausage.

7. Sprinkle cheese over the top and place pizzas in oven.

8. Cook until cheese is melted and bubbly.

* I like to add some fun by making a smiley face on top of the cheese with a strip of red pepper for the mouth and black olives for the eyes.

Makes 6 servings (1 muffin per serving)

Notes

1. R.C. Whitaker and others, "Predicting Obesity in Young Adulthood from Childhood and Parental Obesity," *New England Journal of Medicine* 37 (1997): 869-73.
2. D.S. Freedman and others, "Relationship of Childhood Overweight to Coronary Heart Disease Risk Factors in Adulthood: The Bogalusa Heart Study," *Pediatrics* 108 (2001): 712-18.
3. Ann Harding, "Obese Kids More Likely to Injure Legs, Ankles, Feet," *Reuters Health*, March 1, 2010.
4. "How Does Increased Television Watching 'Weigh Into' Childhood Obesity?" *Science Daily*, October 20, 2005.
5. www.cdc.gov/HealthyYouth/alcoholdrug/index.htm.

For more information on how to bring "The 90-Day Fitness Challenge" live event to your area or to book Phil and Amy Parham for a speaking engagement, please contact them via their website at

www.philandamyfitness.com

Follow them on Twitter **@philandamy**

Become a fan on Facebook at
www.facebook.com/philandamyfitness

Enjoy These Other
Harvest House Books
by Phil and Amy Parham

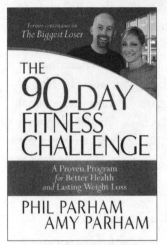

The 90-Day Fitness Challenge
A Proven Program for Better Health and Lasting Weight Loss

Phil and Amy Parham, contestants on NBC's *The Biggest Loser*, provide a faith-based, informative, and motivational book that will encourage those facing weight challenges to permanently transform their lives and live their dreams of being healthier, happier, and more fit.

This is not a diet book for temporary change but a manual for permanent transformation. *The 90-Day Fitness Challenge* will

- encourage readers to embark on a 90-day program for permanent weight loss
- outline simple and practical healthy food and fitness plans
- point the way toward developing better eating habits and an active lifestyle
- incorporate Scripture and faith principles to encourage readers to make God a part of their journey
- provide motivation through heartfelt and encouraging daily readings

The Parhams know from personal experience the obstacles to fitness that overweight readers face. Having lost a combined total of 256 pounds, they come alongside readers to provide inspiration, motivation, and practical life skills on their 90-day journey toward better health and lasting weight loss.

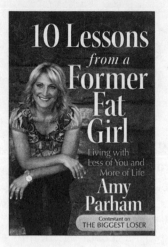

10 Lessons from a Former Fat Girl

Living with Less of You and More of Life

Amy Parham

Amy Parham, a former fat girl who became a fit girl after losing more than 100 pounds, learned what it takes to stay fit inside and out. In *10 Lessons from a Former Fat Girl*, she offers nuggets of insight for changing not only the fat-girl body but also the fat-girl mentality. Focusing on the mental, emotional, and spiritual aspects of our relationship with food and exercise, Amy shows how readers can make this a healthy partnership that brings permanent change. Amy speaks from experience as she

- identifies with the reader struggling with a food addiction
- describes emotional pitfalls that serve as triggers for overeating
- explores the mental and emotional benefits of regular exercise
- illustrates how and why fitness must be a lifelong pursuit
- demonstrates how to transform our minds as well as our bodies

The result is a practical, proven plan that will help any reader reprogram the fat-girl mentality into fit-girl reality.

To learn more about other Harvest House books
or to read sample chapters, log on to our website:

www.harvesthousepublishers.com

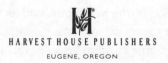

HARVEST HOUSE PUBLISHERS

EUGENE, OREGON